T5-CUL-552

# Hospital-Based Health Promotion Programs for Children and Youth

*An idea generator and guide*
*for marketing services to a growing community*

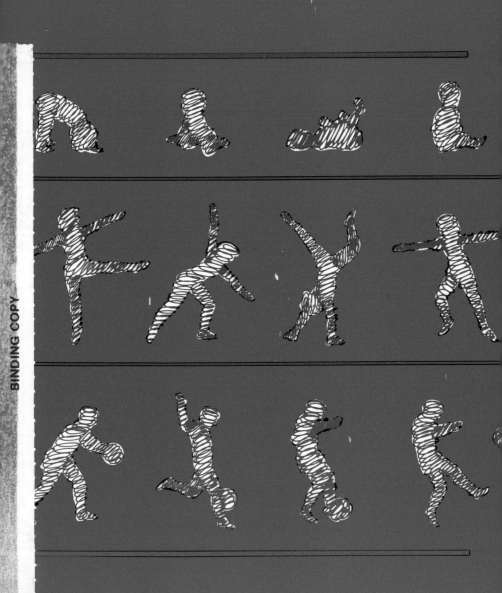

BINDING COPY

By Ruth A. Behrens and Mary E. Longe

# Hospital-Based Health Promotion Programs for Children and Youth

By Ruth A. Behrens and Mary E. Longe

American Hospital Publishing, Inc.,
a wholly owned subsidiary of the
American Hospital Association

WILLIAM MADISON RANDALL LIBRARY UNC AT WILMINGTON

**Library of Congress Cataloging-in-Publication Data**

Behrens, Ruth A.
  Hospital-based health promotion programs for children
and youth.

    "Catalog no. 070189"—P. [4] of cover.
    Includes bibliographies.
    1. Hospitals—Health promotion services.  2. Community
health services for children.  3. Hospitals—United
States—Health promotion services—Case studies.
4. Community health services for children—United States—
Case studies.  I. Longe, Mary E.  II. Title.  [DNLM:
1. Child Health Services—United States.  2. Health
Education—methods—United States.  3. Health Promotion—
methods—United States.  4. Primary Prevention—in infancy
& childhood. WA 320 B421h]
RA975.5.H4B44  1987    362.1'9892        86-28762
ISBN 0-939450-99-2

Catalog no. 070189

© 1987 by American Hospital Publishing, Inc., a wholly owned subsidary of the
American Hospital Association

𝔸ℍ𝔸 is a service mark of the American Hospital Association used under license
by American Hospital Publishing, Inc.

All rights reserved. Reproduction or use of this work in any form or in any information storage and retrieval system is forbidden without the express, written
permission of the publisher.

Printed in the U.S.A.
2.5M-12/86-0168
Text set in 10 point Bookman Light type.

Karen Downing, Editor
Peggy DuMais, Production Coordinator
Marcia Vecchione, Designer
Brian Schenk, Editorial and Acquisitions Manager, Books
Dorothy Saxner, Vice-President, Books

# 1

# Contents

RA975
.5
.H4
.B44
1987

List of Figures . . . . . . . . . . . . . . . . . . . . . . . . . . . . . . . . . . . . . v
Preface . . . . . . . . . . . . . . . . . . . . . . . . . . . . . . . . . . . . . . . . . . vii
Acknowledgments . . . . . . . . . . . . . . . . . . . . . . . . . . . . . . . . . . ix

**Part 1.** Assessing the Need
for Health Promotion Programs for Children . . . . . . . . 1

Chapter 1. Introduction . . . . . . . . . . . . . . . . . . . . . . . . . . . . . 3
Chapter 2. Nondisease Factors Affecting
Children's Health and Safety . . . . . . . . . . . . . . . . . . . . 9
Chapter 3. Lifestyle Factors Affecting Children's Health . . . . . . 23

**Part 2.** Designing Community Health Promotion Programs . . . . 35

Chapter 4. Creative Approaches
to Keeping Children Healthy . . . . . . . . . . . . . . . . . . 37
Chapter 5. Case Study: Alta View Hospital, Sandy, Utah . . . . . 53
Chapter 6. Case Study: Dominican Santa Cruz Hospital,
Santa Cruz, California . . . . . . . . . . . . . . . . . . . . . . . 61

**Part 3.** Designing Health Promotion Programs
for Schools . . . . . . . . . . . . . . . . . . . . . . . . . . . . . . . . . . . . 69

Chapter 7. Schools as Markets
for Health Promotion Programs . . . . . . . . . . . . . . . . 71
Chapter 8. Case Study: Freehold Area Hospital,
Freehold, New Jersey . . . . . . . . . . . . . . . . . . . . . . . 87

**Part 4.** Managing Health Promotion Programs
for Children and Youth . . . . . . . . . . . . . . . . . . . . . . . . . 93

Chapter 9. Making Health Promotion Programs Work
in Your Hospital . . . . . . . . . . . . . . . . . . . . . . . . . . . 95

# List of Figures

Figure 1. Leading Causes of Death
in Children and Young Adults (Ages 1-24) . . . . . . . . 10

Figure 2. U.S. Children, Adolescents, and Young Adults:
Death Rates by Cause, 1982 . . . . . . . . . . . . . . . . . . 11

Figure 3. Causes of Death by Age Groups—1983 Data . . . . . . 12

Figure 4. Suicides per 100,000 Youths, Ages 15-24 . . . . . . . . 18

Figure 5. Suicide Rates, by Sex and Race . . . . . . . . . . . . . . 18

Figure 6. NCYFS Rankings of the 15 Activities
in Physical Education Class
Taking the Largest Portions of Time . . . . . . . . . . . . 26

Figure 7. Rates of Cigarette Smoking
in High School Seniors . . . . . . . . . . . . . . . . . . . . . 27

Figure 8. Percentages of High School Seniors
Who Used Cigarettes Daily . . . . . . . . . . . . . . . . . . 28

Figure 9. Rates of Alcohol Use in High School Seniors . . . . . . 29

# Preface

## Background

The health of children is critical to the future of our communities, our nation, and our world. Without their health, children are unable to experience fully the world created for them. As adults, our task is to provide a safe, nurturing, and healthy environment to help our children grow to their full potential. In 1978, the American Hospital Association established the Center for Health Promotion to help hospitals take a leadership role in ensuring the health of the communities they serve.

Center staff began collecting information about hospital-sponsored health promotion for children and over the years have acted as a liaison between hospitals and national agencies to explore, and in some instances create, initiatives for hospitals to improve and protect the health of children and youth. To further demonstrate its commitment to children's health, AHA established the Center for Women and Children's Health in January 1986. Through the cooperative efforts of these two centers, this publication was created.

The major portion of information for this book was collected from hospitals identified in the 1984 Census of Health Promotion Programs as offering health promotion activities for children of preschool age through high school. All of the hospitals mentioned here have been important to the development of this book. Each has provided information by taking part in phone interviews, submitting documentation of their programming, and subsequently reviewing the material for accuracy. The experiences of these hospitals have provided valuable insights and practical approaches to developing health promotion activities for children and, ultimately, have improved and protected the health of our youth.

## Case Studies

Looking at isolated elements of a community health promotion program for children is one thing; putting the elements together into a successful program that benefits both the hospital and the community is another. Many hospitals have done it well. The three case studies presented in this book were chosen because the institutions have combined a strong commitment to providing health promotion programming for their communities, including children, with top management support, an efficient use of resources, and effective management techniques.

In addition to describing (1) each hospital's setting and environment, (2) the department from which its health promotion programming for children originates, (3) its reasons for targeting children, and (4) an overview of its programming for and about children, each case study examines how the programs are managed. Needs analysis, the planning process, staffing, publicity and promotion, fees and budgets, and evaluation also are discussed for each hospital.

The hospitals examined in the case studies, one with 50 beds, one with 150, one with 250, have produced large programs that have met with an extremely high level of community acceptance. These hospital programs are not described as models to be copied; rather, they are presented in the hope that they will stimulate thinking about various ways in which the selection of staffing and programming, as well as careful application of management principles, can be combined into a successful community health promotion program for children.

In addition to the information contained in the case studies, more details about various aspects of managing these and other programs can be found in this book's final chapter, Making Health Promotion Programs Work in Your Hospital.

# Acknowledgments

Ruth A. Behrens, a consultant based in Washington, DC, was the founding director of the American Hospital Association Center for Health Promotion. Mary E. Longe is the manager of Community Health Promotion and Women's Health, American Hospital Association Centers for Health Promotion and Women's and Children's Health. Both authors are experienced practitioners who have been working with hospitals for many years.

Material for chapters 2 and 3 was contributed by Lloyd J. Kolbe, Ph.D., Acting Chief, School Health and Special Projects, Division of Health Education, Center for Health Promotion and Education, Centers for Disease Control, Atlanta, GA. Shantell Mayberry, American Hospital Association, provided clerical support.

The development of this book is a result of information shared by the following dedicated health promotion professionals.

Shirley Allen, R.N.
Director, Perinatal Nursing
Freeman Hospital
Joplin, MO

Myrna Allums
Health Education Coordinator
Kaiser Foundation Hospital
Martinez, CA

Jacqueline Baird
Director, Health Promotion Wellness Center
Alexandria Hospital
Alexandria, VA

Patricia Brent, M.P.H.
Director of Professional Services
Alice Peck Day Memorial Hospital
Lebanon, NH

Judith A. Brown, R.N.
Health Education Coordinator
Carson City Hospital
Carson City, MI

Joan Christensen
Community Education Coordinator
Cottonwood Hospital
Murray, UT

Robert J. Cole
Vice-President, Human Resources
Riverside Medical Center
Kankakee, IL

Sally Comey, R.N., B.S.
Director, Educational Services
Children's Specialized Hospital
Mountainside, NJ

Brian Cooke
Director, Education and Community Relations
Franciscan Medical Center
Rock Island, IL

Laird P. Covey
Associate Administrator
North Country Hospital
Newport, VT

Roy Cramblit
Personnel Director
Hazel Hawkins Memorial Hospital
Hollister, CA

Diane Cunningham, R.N., M.S.
Assistant Director of Marketing,
    Director of Education
Alta View Hospital
Sandy, UT

Beverly Duffer, R.N., M.S.
Community Education Coordinator
Community Hospitals of Indianapolis
Indianapolis, IN

Rebecca Gannon
Director of Education
St. Luke's Hospital
Davenport, IA

Linda L. Gilstrap
Director, Health Information Center
Bay Hospital Medical Center
Chula Vista, CA

Kim Haithcock
Administrative Director,
    Human Resource Development
Palisades General Hospital
North Bergen, NJ

Cindy Hearrell, R.N.
Cardiac Rehabilitation Coordinator
St. Luke's Hospital
Davenport, IA

Ann M. Hess
Assistant Executive Director, Patient Services
St. John Hospital
Leavenworth, KS

James A. Hruban, H.S.D.
Executive Director
Weller Center for Health Education
Easton Hospital
Easton, PA

Leslie Katz, R.N., M.Ed.
Director, Wellness Center
Freehold Area Hospital
Freehold, NJ

Mary Howe Khan
Community Services Coordinator
Marlborough Hospital
Marlborough, MA

Elaine Leader, Ph.D.
Program Coordinator, Teen Line
Cedars-Sinai Medical Center
Los Angeles, CA

Marilyn LoCicero
Office of Health Education
Central Michigan Community Hospital
Mt. Pleasant, MI

Nancie MacBain
Director, Volunteer Services
Abington Memorial Hospital
Abington, PA

Socorro Macias-Ybarra
Director of Health Promotion
Queen of the Valley Hospital
West Covina, CA

Mary Ann Meidinger
Vice-President, Community Services
MedCenter One, Inc.
Bismarck, ND

Elsie A. Miike, R.N.
Patient Education Coordinator
G.N. Wilcox Memorial Hospital and Health Center
Lihue, HI

David Z. Nareski, R.N., B.S.N.
Development and Community Services Manager
Carson City Hospital
Carson City, MI

Anne Rathke
Patient Educator
Merced Community Medical Center
Merced, CA

Julie E. Santillie
Inservice Coordinator
Mt. Shasta Community Hospital
Mt. Shasta, CA

Shoula Stefos, R.N., M.S.
Chief Administrative Officer
Botsford General Hospital
Farmington Hills, MI

Janet Treftz, M.S.
Health Promotion Coordinator
St. Luke's Hospital
Davenport, IA

Rosemary T. Van Gorder, M.A.
Director, Child Life Program
Orthopaedic Hospital
Los Angeles, CA

Kathleen Ashton Vrabel, M.A.
Child Life and Education Director
Tod Children's Hospital
Youngstown, OH

Nancy Wainer
Director of Public Education
Dominican Santa Cruz Hospital
Santa Cruz, CA

Judy Weink, R.N., M.A.
Community Health Education Coordinator
St. Jude Hospital and Rehabilitation Center
Fullerton, CA

Vicki Wolford, M.A.
Community Health Education Coordinator
Mercy/Memorial Medical Center, Inc.
Benton Harbor, MI

We would like to especially thank the following individuals for their time and effort in reviewing the entire manuscript:

Arnold S. Anderson, M.D.
Member, American Academy of Pediatrics
Minneapolis Children's Medical Center
Minneapolis, MN

Jack Elster
Consultant
Pittsburgh, PA

Beverly Johnson
Executive Director
Association for Care of Children's Health
Washington, DC

Norton Kalishman, M.D.
Medical Director, Community Medicine
Presbyterian Health Care Services
Albuquerque, NM

Elizabeth Lee
Director
Centers for Health Promotion and Women and Children's Health
American Hospital Association
Chicago, IL

Becky Locke-Grosso
Director, Health Promotion
Borgess Medical Center
Kalamazoo, MI

Sandra Long
Director of Wellness
Frankford Hospital
Philadelphia, PA

Philip Nader, M.D.
Division of General Pediatrics
University of California San Diego Medical Center
San Diego, CA

Philip J. Porter, M.D.
Director, Healthy Children
Boston, MA

# Part I

# Assessing the Need for Health Promotion Programs for Children

# 1

# Introduction

## Keeping Children Well:
## An Investment in the Future

It was not many years ago that people scoffed at the thought of hospitals playing a role in keeping people well. After all, hospitals are places people go to get well when they are sick. At one time in their history, hospitals were even places to go to die. But all that has changed.

Today, many hospitals are reexamining, and even rewriting, their missions to clarify and strengthen their roles in maintaining and improving the health of their communities. Some are redefining the business they are in, recognizing that in the past they had engaged in the "illness business" rather than the "health business." Today, these hospitals state confidently that they are in the health business— helping people in their communities regain health when they are sick or injured, helping them maintain good health when they are well, and helping them improve their health at every stage in their lives.

In a climate in which pressures are mounting on all fronts to contain health care costs, hospitals are responding with myriad programs designed to help people stay healthy and out of the hospital. In many hospitals, health promotion has become an integral part of the management of the institution. It contributes significantly to the achievement of hospital goals and therefore must produce the kinds of results desired by the administrators. Communities, too, are coming to expect their hospitals to provide *health care* as well as "illness care."

Hospitals have, indeed, made a commitment to maintaining and improving the health of their communities. It follows, then, that programs designed to help keep children well should, and even must, be considered as a part of their offerings. The studies cited in the following chapters show some alarming statistics about the health problems of our children and youth, as follows:

- As many as half of our children do not engage in regular aerobic activities.
- Eating habits among adolescents are often poor and are being shown to lead to adult health problems.
- Almost 20 percent of all high school seniors smoke cigarettes regularly.
- The use of smokeless tobacco is increasing.
- The percentage of seniors using alcohol daily increased from 1984 to 1985.
- Such problems as child abuse and neglect, suicide, teen pregnancy, and eating disorders are increasing among children and adolescents.

Without a doubt, there is an important role for hospitals in improving the health of the children in their communities. Health promotion staff should carefully examine the data in chapters 2 and 3, investigate which of the problems are most prevalent in their particular community, and decide which problems their hospital is best equipped to address.

When defined narrowly, whatever the audience, health promotion programs are targeted toward well persons, are designed to maintain or improve health and well being, and are voluntary rather than mandatory. Health promotion or wellness topics include physical fitness, nutrition, weight control, stress management, smoking cessation, and alcohol and drug awareness.

In practice, however, most hospital-based health promotion programs go beyond this narrow definition. For example, sick persons may be seen as an audience. Although today's pressure for shorter lengths of stay offers little opportunity for wellness education as part of inpatient care, outpatient programs abound to help those with an illness, injury, or chronic disease reach their greatest potential, given their limitations. Support groups for diabetics and cardiac rehabilitation clinics are just two examples (although in many institutions they would be considered a part of patient education rather than health promotion).

Individuals with existing health conditions or problems who usually are not defined by society as "sick" (overweight adolescents, say, or those with high blood pressure aggravated by stress and poor eating habits) make up another category of potential customers for health promotion programs.

Today, hospital-based health promotion programs also address all aspects of the physical and emotional health of infants, children, and teens, and the range of offerings is growing as hospitals' experiences grow.

More and more, hospitals are including programs for and about youth that deal with social problems and issues in their health promotion offerings. Programs on coping (with divorce, with a new brother or sister), on building self-esteem, and on developing decision-making skills and responsibility illustrate the range of topics that have been added to the basic wellness areas.

Safety, too, has become a staple of most hospital health promotion efforts for children. Teachers, parents, and children themselves often are the target for programs on baby CPR, first aid, and life-saving techniques for choking victims. Bicycle safety rodeos attract as many viewers as riders, but the messages about bike safety come through for all to hear.

## Contributions of Children's Programs to Hospital Goals

Can programs designed to help children stay healthy also help institutions solve such problems as declining census, the need for diversification, underutilization of some services, declining market share, and a lack of name recognition among new residents in the area? The experiences of many hospitals that have put energy and resources into developing programming for children indicate the answer is yes. Although their measurements of these outcomes may be imprecise (it is almost impossible to measure the effect of one program on any of these problems), the administrators of these hospitals believe their offerings for children are making a worthwhile contribution. For instance:

- High-quality health promotion programs aimed at children, or well-designed programs about children directed at parents and teachers, can create considerable good will and positive public relations within a community.
- Through health promotion programs, children can be introduced to hospital staff under positive circumstances, thus helping to alleviate their fears of hospitalization.
- Promotional efforts using newspapers, broadcast media, and even billboards carry the message throughout the area that the hospital cares about the health of its young people and young families.
- Many hospital staff members gain added job satisfaction when given the opportunity to work with children.
- Relationships with other community groups—from voluntary agencies to schools to local business groups—can be solidified and enhanced through cooperative efforts designed to educate children about health.

But efforts aimed at healthy children also have the potential to contribute to more specific, "harder" measures of goal achievement. Following are some of the ways in which health programs for children can have a measurable effect on the hospitals that sponsor them.

## Improvement of Community Health

*High-quality health promotion programs for children will make a significant contribution to improving the health of the community.* Today's children are the adults and parents of tomorrow. They will determine the health status of the communities in which they live as those communities enter the twenty-first century. By teaching infants, children, and teens good health habits while they are young, hospitals may avoid the need to help them adopt new behaviors as adults. The child who learns good nutrition and exercise habits in grade school is less likely to become an obese adult. The teenager who is taught stress management skills and develops strong self-esteem may be less inclined to turn to alcohol or drugs or to become an abusive parent as an adult.

Although many other benefits will emerge as hospitals examine the merits of educating children about primary prevention, this goal of improving the health status of children in the community must remain paramount if the program is to have a significant and lasting impact.

## New Patients for the Hospital

*Health promotion programs for children bring new patients to the hospital.* Orientations, career days, and various classes bring children directly into the hospital; offerings about children, or for parents with children, can introduce the whole family to the hospital. Often these classes bring people into an institution for the first time, and a positive experience can help ensure that they will return the next time they need a hospital.

Programs for children also can introduce them and their parents to individual services the institution offers. Pediatric orientations and prenatal classes (sometimes open to anyone in the community, regardless of which hospital they plan to use) can show off not only services and facilities, but helpful hospital staff as well. New services, such as a freestanding emergency center, can be spotlighted through various programs on safety, handling emergencies, CPR and first aid, and accident-proofing a home for small children. Even underutilized services can benefit from being featured in programs designed to meet the special needs of young families.

These programs sometimes are termed "loss leaders" because they offer a valued educational service at a low cost to attract potential clients into the hospital or to a specific service. Some programs are seen as "case finders" because they may uncover persons with problems who need a hospital's services. But the bottom line must be, first and foremost, to help contribute to improving the physical and emotional health of the target audience.

## New Patients for the Hospital's Doctors

*Programs for children attract new patients for the hospital's doctors.* By spotlighting pediatricians and specialists, health education programs give community residents an opportunity to see physicians in action and to talk with them informally before making a judgment about using them as doctors. For example, an eating disorders specialist might give a free evening lecture on anorexia nervosa and bulimia, or a pediatrician could present a workshop on parent-child communications.

## Competitive Edge for the Hospital

*Programs for children give a hospital a competitive edge.* More and more, patients are playing a role in selecting their hospitals. Thus it is increasingly important that potential patients be familiar with a hospital's name. The promotional campaign used to alert the public to programs for children also serves to make them aware of that hospital's name, over and over. Any publicity generated following a health promotion activity, such as the newspaper story about a young girl who saved a baby's life because of CPR skills learned in a hospital-sponsored babysitting class, will reinforce the name recognition and, in this example, the name also will be associated with a high-quality program. Those who personally have had positive experiences attending health education classes will find it an easy mental leap from associating the institution with high-quality health education to associating it with high-quality health care. To carry the comparison even further, the fact that a family member has been to a hospital for a health education program may mean that he or she has met at least one staff member and thus already "knows" someone there. When put together, all these elements can contribute to a hospital having a strong competitive edge over its neighbors.

## Testing Mechanism for New Markets

*Programs for children are an excellent mechanism for testing new markets*—for a new institution, a new service, or a new satellite site. Several hospitals have had success offering a series of health education programs in an area where they were considering establishing a new service. By running a series of sports medicine clinics, one hospital was able to test the market for a new sports medicine center. A series of wellness programs for women and children in a shopping mall served as a useful test for a new women's and children's hospital.

# Goals of This Book

*Hospital-Based Health Promotion Programs for Children and Youth* is designed to encourage and assist hospitals in providing more effective health promotion programming for children of all ages. It provides background data on the health of our nation's youth, information that can help hospitals make responsible, informed decisions about the types of programs to implement. In addition, it explores the scope and depth of current hospital-based activities in order to give hospital personnel an overview of which programs are working in other communities, how they work, and how to start similar ones if that is the hospital's choice.

It is the authors' hope that hospital staff, using the information and case studies in this book, can work with their communities to develop programs that are appropriate, cost-effective, and beneficial to hospitals as well as to the communities they serve.

# 2

## Nondisease Factors Affecting Children's Health and Safety

To help program developers make informed decisions about hospital-based *health promotion* programs for healthy children, rather than *patient education or disease prevention* programs, this chapter examines some of the major nondisease indicators affecting the health and safety of today's children and adolescents.

One should note that a variety of factors affect the health of children. These include the traditional measures of health (such as heredity, health of family members and peers, race, mother's level of prenatal care), socioeconomic circumstances (such as family income, availability of health services, living conditions, and place of residence—inner city, rural, and so forth), and, of course, the individual's own lifestyle habits. Hereditary factors are beyond the control of any person; socioeconomic factors are beyond the control of children, by virtue of their age and lack of power; but the individual behaviors that contribute to good health can be controlled even by very young children. These behaviors are discussed in chapter 3.

An in-depth examination of many of the above-mentioned factors, such as socioeconomic circumstances and heredity, is beyond the scope of this publication. However, because they are so all-pervasive, and because hospital staff, parents, and teachers need to be aware of them and may be able to address them in programs about children directed to adults, some factors will be touched on as they relate to specific health problems.

This chapter discusses some of the major preventable nondisease causes of poor health, injury, or death in children and adolescents:

- Accidents
- Motor vehicle accidents
- Child abuse and neglect
- Teenage pregnancy
- Obesity

- Eating disorders
- Suicide

Each section that deals with one of the above topics includes current data and information in an attempt to help hospitals determine which problems are most important in their communities and on which areas their institution could have the greatest impact.

In addition, some information is provided concerning hospital use by children. Even hospitals without pediatric units can expect to admit children as patients occasionally. Information about trends in their hospitalization may be useful in alerting key decision makers to the importance of this audience as current and potential clients.

## Causes of Poor Health, Injury, and Death among Children

Although the focus of this book is on healthy children, it is important when discussing health promotion to be aware of the effect of lifestyle on diseases and other causes of death and injury. It is difficult to get good data on leading causes of illness and injury among children; however, good information is available on mortality. Following is a list of the leading causes of death among children and adolescents in the United States, along with those risk factors that can be related to them (see figures 1 and 2). Although this information probably will not be the sole driving force behind selecting hospital-based health promotion activities for children and youth, it can be a valuable part of any decision-making process.

When one looks at the causes of death among children and young people, broken down by smaller age groups, and when actual numbers of deaths in each category are included, the results look somewhat different (see figure 3).

| Leading Causes | Associated Risk Factors |
| --- | --- |
| 1. Motor Vehicle Accidents | Alcohol, seat belts, driving speed |
| 2. Other Accidents | Alcohol, smoking (fire), home hazards, handgun availability |
| 3. Homicide | Handgun availability, alcohol, drugs, stress |
| 4. Suicide | Handgun availability, alcohol, drugs, stress |
| 5. Cancer | Smoking, alcohol, solar radiation, diet, environmental pollution |
| 6. Heart Disease | Smoking, high blood pressure, elevated serum cholesterol (diet), obesity, lack of exercise |

**Figure 1.   Leading Causes of Death in Children and Young Adults (ages 1-24)**

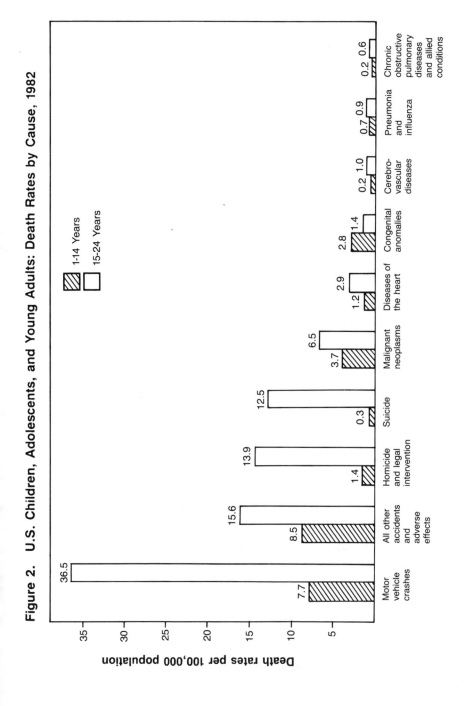

Figure 2. U.S. Children, Adolescents, and Young Adults: Death Rates by Cause, 1982

**Ages 1–4**

| Cause of Death | Number of Deaths |
|---|---|
| 1. All accidents | 3,043 |
|   1a. Motor vehicle | (1,043) |
|   1b. Other accidents | (2,000) |
| 2. Congenital anomalies | 913 |
| 3. Cancer | 654 |
| 4. Diseases of the heart | 349 |
| 5. Homicide | 320 |
| 6. Influenza and pneumonia | 232 |
| Total reported deaths, 1983 | 7,801 |

**Ages 5–14**

| Cause of Death | Number of Deaths |
|---|---|
| 1. All Accidents | 4,321 |
|   1a. Motor vehicle | (2,241) |
|   1b. Other accidents | (2,080) |
| 2. Cancer | 1,318 |
| 3. Congenital anomalies | 471 |
| 4. Homicide | 357 |
| 5. Diseases of the heart | 318 |
| 6. Suicide | 205 |
| Total reported deaths, 1983 | 9,143 |

**Ages 15–24**

| Cause of Death | Number of Deaths |
|---|---|
| 1. All Accidents | 19,756 |
|   1a. Motor vehicle | (14,289) |
|   1b. Other accidents | (5,467) |
| 2. Homicide | 5,037 |
| 3. Suicide | 4,845 |
| 4. Cancer | 2,293 |
| 5. Diseases of the heart | 1,068 |
| 6. Congenital anomalies | 554 |
| Total reported deaths | 39,082 |

**Figure 3.   Causes of Death by Age Groups—1983 Data**

## Accidents

During 1980-81, more than 14 million days of school per year were lost to children because of injuries. This amounted to 36.2 days per 100 children per year. Analysis of these lost school days for children ages 6 to 16 years shows the following:[1]

- The rate of school days lost was higher for boys than girls, 43.6 to 28.5 days lost, respectively, per 100 children per year.

- Children in standard metropolitan statistical area (SMSA) central cities had a higher rate of school-loss days than children from other areas.
- Children from the lowest-income families (less than $10,000 a year) had a very high rate of school-loss days because of injuries—66.3 per 100 children.
- The rate of school-loss days was higher among black children than white children—49.5 days per 100 children versus 34.7 days, respectively.
- The highest rates of school-loss days were attributed to accidents occurring at home, at school, and on streets and highways, in that order.

Accidents affected more than school days lost among children. Motor vehicle accidents and all other accidents rank as the number one and number two killers of children. Taken together, they are a formidable threat to the lives of our children.

- Visits to emergency rooms as a result of accidents were highest among the under-6 age group, followed by the 6-to-16 age group and the 17-to-24 age group.[1]
- Almost 62 percent of all children injured in the under-6 age group were hurt in or at their homes.[1]
- In 1982, non-motor-vehicle accidents accounted for 10 percent of all deaths from infancy through the teenage years.[2,3]
- For all age groups except under 1 year, drownings account for the highest fatality from non-motor-vehicle accidents, with burns and fires second.[3]
- Among children under 1 year, non-motor-vehicle death rates are highest for burns and fires, followed by drownings and falls.[3]
- Accidents account for about 45 percent of all childhood deaths. Of these, motor vehicle accidents are responsible for more than 20 percent of the deaths, drownings for 8 percent, and fires for 6 percent.[4]

Of special interest to hospitals is the fact that at least one in every five children requires hospital treatment each year for injuries suffered in bicycle spills, kitchen burns, and other accidental tumbles and hazards. In a study conducted in Massachussetts and published in 1984 in the *American Journal of Public Health,* falls, often down stairs, were the most commonly reported accidents, followed by sports injuries, being struck by an object, and being cut or jabbed. Infants and older teenagers were most prone to injuries, and boys had more mishaps, according to the study.[5]

The U.S. Consumer Product Safety Commission (CPSC) estimates that 126,000 toy-related injuries were treated in U.S. hospital emergency rooms in 1984. Of these, about 80 percent were to children under 15 years. Riding toys (not including bicycles) were associated with more injuries than any other type of toy. Other types of toys frequently reported as being associated with injuries were flying toys, toy weapons, toy boxes or chests, models, toy sports equipment, and crayons or chalk. The CPSC received reports of 33 toy-related deaths in 1984. The ingestion and aspiration of balloons, small toys, such as balls and marbles, or parts of toys, such as the eye from a stuffed animal, were associated with 15 fatalities, including 9 children under 3 years of age. Tricycles and other riding toys were associated with 8 fatalities to children 4 years old or younger who rode into pools or into the paths of vehicles.[6]

## Motor Vehicle Accidents

Consistently, the highest rate of death in motor vehicle accidents is among the 15-to-24 age group (35.1 deaths per 100,000 resident population in 1983). White males in this age group experienced the highest rate, 57 deaths per 100,000 population, followed by black males (28.3 per 100,000), white females (18.8 per 100,000), and black females (8.6 per 100,000).[7] Rates for children under 15 are not nearly as high, due in some part to the increased use of infant car restraints (see chapter 3, Lifestyle Factors Affecting Children's Health; Seat Belts). There were 5.2 deaths in motor vehicle accidents per 100,000 population for children under 1 year, 7.5 for those 1 to 4 years old, and 6.6 for those 5 to 14.[7]

During 1982, 22.5 percent of all motor vehicle deaths were to children 19 years old and younger,[8] and constituted the leading cause of death for this age group.[3] One out of five deaths for those 1 to 15 years old, and two of every five deaths for those 15 to 19, were caused by motor vehicle accidents in 1983.[2,3]

## Child Abuse and Neglect

In recent years, the problems of child abuse and neglect have been brought to the attention of virtually all Americans, largely through the public media. Many would suggest that the nation is witnessing an epidemic, even though it is impossible to accurately document all abuse and neglect cases.

At this time, the best available source of data is the National Study on Child Neglect and Abuse Report, a project conducted since 1974 by a division of the American Humane Association. The study, funded through the National Center of Child Abuse and Neglect of the U.S. Department of Health and Human Services, gathers its information from official reports of child maltreatment documented by child protective services (CPS) agencies nationwide.[9]

Among the findings of the 1984 study are the following:

- There were 1,726,649 abused or maltreated children reported nationwide in 1984. This represents an increase of 17 percent since 1983 and an increase of 158 percent since 1976.
- The rate of reporting has shown an even larger increase, from 10.1 abused or neglected children for every 1,000 children in 1976, to a reported 27.3 abused or neglected children per 1,000 in 1984.
- This increase in reporting does not yet approach the number of actual child victims estimated through survey research. A 1985 analysis based on the Louis Harris survey methods suggests there were 1.5 million children subjected to severe physical violence within their families in 1985. This is 7 times the number reported as physically injured by CPS agencies nationwide.[3,10]
- Although neglect still constitutes 58 percent of total reporting, it is declining in proportion to abuse as a percentage of all reporting. However, this decrease is only relative; total reportings of neglect, as well as abuse, are rising.
- Half of all abuse reports still come from nonprofessionals (friends, neighbors, relatives, self: 36.2 percent; anonymous: 12.4 percent; other sources: 1.9 percent), although the percentage of reports coming from professionals has risen from 46 percent in 1981 to 49.6 percent in 1984.
- The average age of the involved child is 7.
- However, 43 percent of the children reported were under 6.
- Slightly more female than male children are reported as abused or neglected.
- Almost half of the families reported were receiving public assistance.
- 37 percent of the families reported had a single female caretaker.
- There has been a 35 percent increase in sexual abuse reports between 1983 and 1984.
- Of the 1984 reported cases of child maltreatment, 67 percent of the children were white, 20.8 percent black, 9.6 percent Hispanic, and 2.6 percent were other races.

## Teenage Pregnancy

Infants born to teenage mothers are at an increased risk of dying before they reach their first birthdays and are known to have twice the normal rate of low birth weight.[11] Young maternal age may also be a predictor of sudden infant death, gastrointestinal problems, and accidents in infancy. Later in life, children born to teenage mothers are less likely to adapt well at school, are more likely to score low on IQ tests, and have an increased risk of repeating at least one grade in school. There also is some evidence that children born to young mothers have an increased risk of neglect, mental retardation, congenital defects, and other handicapping conditions such as epilepsy.[3]

Teenage mothers also face adverse health and social consequences, but it is believed that many of the health consequences (such as iron deficiency anemia and complications of toxemia) are more a function of socioeconomic conditions than of biological factors.[3]

Teenage pregnancy has important implications for both the mother and the infant.

- In 1983, 13.7 percent of all live births were to girls under age 20. More than one-third of these births, or 182,405 infants, were to mothers aged 17 or under.[3,12]
- In 1983, the birth rate for girls aged 15 to 17 was 32.0 per 100; for girls aged 10 to 14, the rate was 1.1 per 100.[3,13]
- Although births to teenage mothers constituted only 13.7 percent of all live births in 1983, these babies accounted for almost 20 percent of all low-birth-weight infants in the nation.[3,13]
- Teenage mothers are more likely to be unmarried, have lower educational attainment, have less prenatal care, and give birth to a larger percentage of low-birth-weight infants than mothers in their twenties.[7]
- Among pregnant women under age 20, one in nine received little or no prenatal care.[12]
- 25 percent of the infants born to mothers under age 14 are premature, a rate 3 times higher than that of older mothers.[3,14]
- In 1983, 14.5 percent of births to girls under 15 and 10.5 percent of births to girls 15 to 17 were low birth weight, as compared to 5.9 percent for women aged 25 to 29.
- In 1983, high percentages of black, Puerto Rican, American Indian, and Mexican infants were born to teenage mothers (25, 22, 22, and 18 percent, respectively).[7]
- Among white mothers, 12 percent of births were to teenagers; among Cubans, 9 percent of births were to teenagers. The percentage was much lower for Asian-Americans, with just 1 percent of Chinese, 3 percent of Japanese, and 6 percent of Filipino infants born to teenage mothers.[7]

## Obesity

An analysis of data from recent Health and Nutrition Examination Surveys (HANES), which are conducted every three to four years by the National Center for Health Statistics, revealed that the prevalence of obesity among 6-to-11-year-old U.S. children increased by 54 percent in the past 15 to 20 years. The prevalence of obesity increased by 39 percent among 12-to-17-year-olds as well. For some groups of children, the picture is even worse. The prevalence of obesity increased by almost twice the amount in preadolescent black children as it did in preadolescent whites.[15]

Obesity in childhood does have implications for adult health, according to a researcher at the Western Psychiatric Institute and Clinic, Pittsburgh.[15] Forty percent of children who are obese at age 7 become obese adults. Seventy percent of obese adolescents become obese adults.

On the basis of three studies, a researcher at the New England Medical Center Hospitals, Boston, concluded that "next to prior obesity, television viewing is the strongest predictor of subsequent obesity because (1) children eat more while watching TV; (2) they eat more of the foods advertised on TV (often junk foods); (3) television gives the message that you can eat and be thin (nearly everyone on television is thin); and (4) watching television is inactive."[15]

## Eating Disorders

In recent years, both anorexia nervosa and bulimia have become serious health problems, especially among young women. According to a study conducted among sophomores in four California high schools,[16] one in eight 10th-graders tries to lose weight by vomiting or using laxatives or other drugs. Although few could be diagnosed as being true bulimics, 13 percent admitted to at least occasional use of self-induced vomiting, laxatives, or diuretics (which increase urine output). Twice as many girls as boys used purging to lose weight. Most of this so-called purging behavior occurred monthly or less often, according to a report on the study in the *Journal of the American Medical Association*,[16] and few students used such methods as often as once a week.

According to the study director, "What's alarming is that at age 15 we see kids beginning to use some of these unhealthy weight regulation strategies that, if unchecked, may develop into full-blown eating disorders."

Bulimia can result in such potentially fatal problems as stomach rupture, heart attack, and abnormal heart rhythm. Other complications include serious dental problems, disruption of the menstrual cycle, and inflammation, laceration, or rupturing of the esophagus. Researchers have not ascertained why some persons develop bulimia, but many have said that thinness has been linked to beauty, success, and happiness in modern times. That may trigger extreme dieting measures, even in some thin persons who perceive themselves as overweight.

The study director suggests that it is important to work with adolescents on weight control, to focus on eating healthily and increasing physical activity. He also suggests that school health classes should include information on eating disorders.

## Suicide

Suicide among young persons has become a serious national concern in recent years; in some communities the numbers of teen suicides and suicide attempts has caused widespread concern.

In 1983, the most recent year for which data are available, there were 205 reported suicides among children 5 to 14 years old. In the 15-to-24 group, 4,845 young persons killed themselves,[3,8] representing the third highest cause of death in this age group. Suicide rates in this latter group increased steadily from 1960 to 1979, but have been dropping slightly since then (see figure 4).[7]

However, suicide rates per 1,000 in this group differ dramatically by sex and race, with the rate for white males being almost double the next nearest group, black males. Rates for all groups increased from 1982 to 1983 (see figure 5).[6]

| Year | Suicides per 100,000 |
|------|----------------------|
| 1950 | 4.5 |
| 1960 | 5.2 |
| 1970 | 8.8 |
| 1979 | 12.4 |
| 1980 | 12.3 |
| 1981 | 12.3 |
| 1982 | 12.1 |
| 1983 | 11.9 |

**Figure 4.  Suicides per 100,000 Youths, Ages 15–24**

| Year | White Males | Black Males | White Females | Black Females |
|------|-------------|-------------|---------------|---------------|
| 1980 | 21.4 | 12.3 | 4.6 | 2.3 |
| 1981 | 21.1 | 11.1 | 4.9 | 2.4 |
| 1982 | 21.2 | 11.0 | 4.5 | 2.2 |
| 1983 | 20.6 | 11.5 | 4.6 | 2.7 |

**Figure 5.  Suicide Rates, by Sex and Race**

## Hospital Use by Children

Most hospitals, even those without pediatric units, occasionally admit children. Analysis of hospital- and area-specific diagnoses for which children are hospitalized can provide additional insight into the factors influencing their health. The following national data may highlight areas in which individual communities differ from the average, possibly denoting health problems of special concern.

Seventy-one of every 1,000 children under age 15 in 1982 were discharged from a nonfederal, short-stay hospital; 25 of the 71 were surgery patients. The average length of stay for those in this age group was 4.6 days, with surgery patients staying an average of 4.7 days. For every 1,000 males under 15 years, 79.9 were discharged from a hospital. Following is a breakdown of the diagnoses for which they were admitted: 5.2, acute respiratory infections; 5.1, chronic diseases of the tonsils and adenoids; 4.0, congenital anomalies; 3.7, otitis media and eustachian tube disorders; 3.8, fractures.[7]

For every 1,000 females under age 15 in 1982, 62.0 were discharged from a hospital following these diagnoses: 5.8, chronic diseases of the tonsils and adenoids; 4.9, pneumonia; 2.7, congenital anomalies; 2.5, otitis media and eustachian tube disorders. The rates of discharge for all causes for both males and females decreased from 1981 to 1982.[7]

The poorer the family, the more likely children in that family are to have no regular source of care, and to have a place, rather than a regular physician, as their source of care.[17] Children in poor families covered by Medicaid frequently use hospital outpatient departments as their regular source of care.[18] Even though poor children experience far more illness than non-poor children, they receive health care services far less frequently.[19] Hospitals that are aware of poor children's needs and the above-mentioned behavior patterns can perhaps address those needs through programs in schools and in the community *before* health concerns become full-fledged problems.

## Conclusion

In identifying problems that can be affected by health promotion, hospitals traditionally look at diseases. But to limit thinking in this manner when planning programs for children overlooks some of today's most urgent health issues: teen pregnancies, suicides, eating disorders, child abuse, and others. Certainly, most hospitals will begin their programs for children with activities that are enjoyable and of the most immediate interest to young audiences. But the institutions with a serious commitment to keeping children well will recognize that, in order to make a lasting difference within their communities, these more complex physical and emotional issues must be addressed as well.

# References

1. National Center for Health Statistics. Persons injured and disabled days due to injuries, United States, 1980-81. *Vital Health Statistics.* Series 10, No.149 DHHS Pub. No. (PHS)85-1577. Washington, DC: U.S. Government Printing Office, Mar. 1985.

2. National Center for Health Statistics. Advance report of final mortality statistics, 1982. *Monthly Vital Statistics Report 33 (20 Dec).* Supplement. DHHS Pub. No. (PHS)85-1120. Washington, DC: U.S. Government Printing Office, 1984.

3. Miller, G.A., and others. *Monitoring Children's Health: Key Indicators.* Washington, DC: American Public Health Association, 1986.

4. U.S. Department of Health, Education, and Welfare. *Healthy People: The Surgeon General's Report on Health Promotion and Disease Prevention.* DHEW Pub. No. (PHS)79-55071. Washington, DC: U.S. Government Printing Office, 1979.

5. Gallagher, S., and others. The incidence of injuries among 87,000 Massachusetts children and adolescents: Surveillance system. *American Journal of Public Health,* 1984 74(12):1340-47.

6. U.S. Consumer Product Safety Commission. *Toy-Related Injury Data Update, 1985.* Washington, DC: USCPSC, Nov. 1985.

7. National Center for Health Statistics. *Health—United States, 1985.* Washington, DC: Department of Health and Human Services, 1984.

8. National Highway Traffic Safety Administration. *Fatal Accident Reporting System, 1982.* DOT Pub. No. (HS)806-142. Washington, DC: Department of Transportation, 1984.

9. American Humane Association. *Highlights of Official Child Neglect and Abuse Reporting, 1984.* Denver, CO: American Association for Protecting Children, AHA, 1985.

10. Gelles, R.J., and Strauss, M.A. *Is Violence Toward Children Increasing: A Comparison of 1975 and 1985 National Survey Rates.* Durham, NH: Family Violence Research Program, 1985.

11. U.S. Department of Health and Human Services. *Surgeon General's Workshop on Maternal and Infant Health.* DHHS Pub. No. (PHS)81-50161. Washington, DC: U.S. Government Printing Office, 1981.

12. Children's Defense Fund. *A Children's Defense Budget.* Washington, DC: CDF, 1986.

13. National Center for Health Statistics. Advance report of final natality statistics, 1983. *Monthly Vital Statistics Report 34 (Sept).* Supplement. DHHS Pub. No. (PHS)85-1120. Washington, DC: U.S. Government Printing Office, 1985.

14. Petit, M., and Overcash, D. *America's Children: Powerless and in Need of Powerful Friends. A 1983 Status Report to the National Governors' Association.* Augusta, ME: Maine Department of Public Health, 1983.

15. Kolata, G. Obese children: A growing problem. *Science,* 1986 Apr. 4 232:20-21.

16. Killen, J.D., and others. Self-induced vomiting and laxative and diuretic use among teenagers. *Journal of the American Medical Association,* 1986 255(11):1447-49.

17. National Center for Health Statistics. Hospital use by children: United States, 1983. *NCHS Advancedata,* 1985 109(1):51.

18. Kovar, M., and Meny, D. A statistical profile *in* Select panel for the promotion of child health. *Better Health for Our Children,* vol. 3. Washington, DC: U.S. Department of Health and Human Services, 1980.

19. Kovar, M. Health status of U.S. children and use of medical care. *Public Health Reports,* 1982 97:3-15.

# 3

# Lifestyle Factors Affecting Children's Health

Although conclusive scientific data do not exist to prove that many positive lifestyle habits engaged in during youth actually prevent adult diseases, common sense tells us that good health behaviors established early in life are likely to be continued to adulthood. So although it cannot be proven that children who eat low-fat diets and engage in vigorous, regular physical activity will have fewer heart attacks than those who do not, it can be hoped that at least some of those good habits will be sustained over the years, thereby building up a lifetime of positive health behaviors. There also is reason to believe that the longer an individual delays taking up poor health habits, such as smoking or using alcohol to excess, the more likely he or she will be to shun them forever.

It is for these reasons (the likelihood that good health habits established in youth will become part of adult lifestyles, and that bad habits, if postponed during childhood and adolescence, will not be tempting in adulthood) that hospitals are investing resources in encouraging children and adolescents to lead healthy lives.

But just how healthy are today's children? Is the job of promoting good health among the young already being done? In order to help hospitals assess the health of their young persons, a brief overview of selected lifestyle factors follows. In some cases, little or no conclusive information exists. In others, patterns can clearly be seen. The information is presented so that hospitals can identify issues that need further investigation as they assess the health status of youth in their own communities and make decisions about what kinds of programs and services would be useful at the local level.

Because of the changing composition of today's family, this chapter also looks at the increase in the percentage of mothers who work. This factor is important not only because of the direct effect it may have on the health of children, but also because of its importance relative to such indirect issues as identifying program topics (latch-key children, home safety, loneliness, babysitting, and so forth) and scheduling programs for children.

## Nutrition

Although serious morbidity and mortality related to poor nutrition are uncommon in this country, 1983 data from the Nationwide Food Consumption Survey show that over 45 percent of the 4-to-7-year-olds and 1-to-4-year-olds fell below the recommended daily allowances for calcium, and 30 percent of the 4-to-7-year-olds and 90 percent of the 1-to-4-year-olds fell below the recommended level for iron. Vitamin B6 was low in 42 percent and 20 percent, respectively, and vitamin C was low in 35 percent and 21 percent, respectively.[1]

However, nutrition problems are more prevalent among poor children. The Massachusetts Department of Public Health found that 10,000 to 17,500 poor children in that state suffered stunted growth, largely due to chronic malnutrition. Nearly one in five low-income children studied was either stunted, anemic, or abnormally underweight.[2]

Adolescents exhibit a variety of eating behaviors that cause concern. These include skipping meals; snacking, especially on sweets; frequently eating fast foods; choosing unconventional foods for certain meals; and dieting sporadically. Although in general youths now exhibit remarkable growth, certain specific nutrition-related adolescent disorders do warrant attention, including obesity (10 to 20 percent of adolescents have high rates of anxiety about their weight), alcohol abuse, anorexia nervosa, bulimia, low iron intake, and high fat consumption beyond the end of adolescence.[3] In addition, there are serious dental risks related to poor nutrition.

High fat consumption may raise the risk of coronary heart disease. Although there are no longitudinal (long-term) data to establish that having high cholesterol levels in childhood increases the risk of coronary heart disease in adulthood, many authors cite extensive indirect evidence of such a relationship.[4]

## Physical Fitness

Two recent studies underscore the fact that as many as half of the nation's children and youth are not engaging in appropriate physical activities (that is, activities that provide cardiovascular conditioning) and that levels of fitness have not improved in the past ten years.

The National Children and Youth Fitness Study (NCYFS), conducted by the U.S. Office of Disease Prevention and Health Promotion (Department of Health and Human Services), was designed to determine how fit and how active 5th- through 12th-grade students actually are.[5] One of the most important measurements attempted to determine how many youngsters were engaging in appropriate physical activity. Almost 60 percent of those surveyed reported that they believed they took part in vigorous physical activities, yet just 41 percent reported regular experiences of sweating and breathing hard during exercise. Thus, drawing from this self-reported data, it appears that approximately half of the American children and youth in grades 5 through 12 do not perform the minimum weekly requirement of vigorous physical activity needed to maintain an effectively functioning cardiorespiratory system.

Further, seasonality in exercise patterns, due to the inability of children to shift physical activities from one season to the next or to perpetuate activities despite changes in seasons, frequently results in their failing to receive appropriate physical activity year round. Greater emphasis needs to be placed on finding options for, and establishing the acceptability of, vigorous physical activity in all four seasons.

The study also questioned students about their physical activities outside formal physical education classes. Boys and girls in three age groups (grades 5 and 6; 7, 8, and 9; and 10, 11, and 12) were asked to rank activities according to which took the greatest portion of their time. Only two activities for boys (bicycling and football) and three for girls (calisthenics/exercise, disco or popular dance, and swimming) ranked in the top four across all three grade groups. The findings of this portion of the study (see figure 6) provide useful information for hospitals considering developing physical fitness programs for students in the middle and upper grades.[5]

The 1985 School Population Fitness Survey conducted for the President's Council on Physical Fitness concluded that the performance of youth in 1985 was not much different from that of youth in 1975.[6] There was still a low level of performance in important components of physical fitness by millions of our youth, especially on cardiorespiratory (heart-lung) endurance tests. This is especially distressing because many experts are calling heart disease a pediatric disease, the conditions that relate to these problems are developing in so many of our youth.

The study also concluded that:
- There is poor performance by large numbers of boys and girls on tests of arm and shoulder muscle strength and endurance. This is important because many of today's youth have insufficient strength to handle their own body weight in case of emergency and often are unable to carry on daily work or recreational activities successfully and safely.
- The large number of boys and girls who perform at low levels in sit-ups and the sit-and-reach test portend adults with back

| Physical Activity | Grades 5, 6 | | Grades 7, 8, 9 | | Grades 10, 11, 12 | |
|---|---|---|---|---|---|---|
| | Boys | Girls | Boys | Girls | Boys | Girls |
| Badminton | * | * | * | * | 10 | 10 |
| Baseball/Softball | 6 | 6 | 3 | 5 | 3 | 4 |
| Basketball | 3 | 3 | 1 | 1 | 1 | 2 |
| Calisthenics/Exercises | 1 | 1 | 2 | 2 | 5 | 3 |
| Climbing ropes | 13 | 15 | * | * | * | * |
| Aerobic dance | * | 15 | * | 9 | * | 6 |
| Dodgeball/Bombardment | 5 | 9 | 9 | 13 | 15 | * |
| Field hockey/Street hockey | * | * | 13 | * | 14 | * |
| Football—tackle | * | * | * | * | 12 | * |
| Football—touch | 11 | 13 | 4 | 8 | 6 | 7 |
| Gymnastics—apparatus | * | * | * | * | * | 15 |
| Gymnastics—free exercise | * | 13 | * | 15 | * | 13 |
| Gymnastics—tumbling | 14 | 12 | * | 11 | * | 12 |
| Jogging | 2 | 2 | 5 | 4 | 7 | 5 |
| Jumping or skipping rope | 12 | 10 | 14 | 13 | * | 13 |
| Kickball | 4 | 4 | 12 | 7 | * | 15 |
| Relays | 7 | 5 | 10 | 11 | * | * |
| Running sprints | 9 | 10 | 8 | 9 | 13 | * |
| Soccer | 7 | 6 | 7 | 6 | 8 | 7 |
| Swimming | * | * | * | * | 9 | 15 |
| Tag | 15 | * | * | * | — | — |
| Tennis | * | * | * | * | 11 | 11 |
| Volleyball | 9 | 8 | 6 | 3 | 2 | 1 |
| Weight lifting or training | * | * | 10 | * | 4 | 9 |
| Wrestling | * | * | 14 | * | * | — |

* Activity was performed, but did not enter the top 15 for a grade/sex cell.
— Activity was not performed by a grade/sex cell.

**Figure 6.   NCYFS Rankings of the 15 Activities in Physical Education Class Taking the Largest Portions of Time.**

problems, one of America's leading health problems in the workplace.

- Girls declined or stayed at the same level in their performance on eight of the nine test items after age 14. The one test they continued to improve on when older was the sit-and-reach test of flexibility.
- Boys performed better than girls on every test of physical fitness except flexibility.

Because physical fitness has been shown to be significantly related to the ability to do physical activities such as household chores, work, sports, and dance, in an effective and safe manner, the fitness level of youth is an important concern for any institution that has a commitment to promoting the health of children.

## Smoking

Very little reliable data are available on the cigarette smoking habits of adolescents, but a 1985 survey of more than 16,000 high school seniors from public and private schools showed an increase among "daily users" over 1984, while those having "used in the past month" has not declined significantly since 1980.[7]

Female seniors have consistently smoked more cigarettes than male seniors since 1976, according to the High School Senior Drug Use Survey,[7] although both groups declined from 1983 to 1984 (most recent data available). The survey, which has been conducted yearly since 1975, reveals generally declining rates of cigarette smoking among high school seniors for most of that period (see figure 7).

| Year | Percent Who Used in Past Month | Percent Who Use Daily |
|------|--------------------------------|------------------------|
| 1975 | 37.0 | 26.9 |
| 1977 | 38.0 | 28.8 |
| 1979 | 34.0 | 27.5 |
| 1981 | 29.0 | 20.3 |
| 1983 | 30.0 | 21.2 |
| 1984 | 29.0 | 18.7 |
| 1985 | 30.0 | 19.5 |

**Figure 7.   Rates of Cigarette Smoking in High School Seniors**

The difference in smoking rates between males and females continues to be dramatic, as demonstrated in figure 8. The pattern of high school females smoking more heavily than males appears to be carrying over into smoking patterns of adults as well. Smoking rates are decreasing for all groups except women between ages 20 and 24; and lung cancer has now replaced breast cancer as the leading cause of death among women.

## Smokeless Tobacco

The use of smokeless tobacco by young persons is being increasingly recognized as a problem. A Louisiana study, the Bogalusa Heart

| | Percent | |
|---|---|---|
| **Year** | **Males** | **Females** |
| 1975 | 26.9 | 26.4 |
| 1977 | 27.1 | 30.0 |
| 1979 | 22.3 | 27.8 |
| 1981 | 18.1 | 21.7 |
| 1983 | 19.2 | 22.2 |
| 1984 | 16.0 | 20.5 |

**Figure 8.   Percentages of High School Seniors Who Used Cigarettes Daily**

Study, suggests that the use of smokeless tobacco may be rising among adolescent boys as cigarette smoking declines.[8] A recent report of the U.S. Department of Health and Human Services indicates that 70 percent of young male users of smokeless tobacco regard it as more acceptable than, or as acceptable as, cigarette smoking.[9]

The same survey reported that 16 percent of males between ages 12 and 25 have used some form of smokeless tobacco within the past year, and that from one-third to one-half of these used it at least once a week. Use by females of all ages is consistently less than for males, with about 2 percent using smokeless tobacco in the past year. One study found that the average age of first use was 10 years old, with regular and daily use starting as early as age 12.[8] Fifty percent cited "pressure from friends" as their primary reason for initiating use, but continued use was most often attributed to enjoyment of taste (64 percent) and habit strength or "being hooked" (37 percent).

State and local studies corroborate these national findings. The prevalence of smokeless tobacco use by youth and young adults varies widely by region, but use is not limited to a single region. In several parts of the country, use of smokeless tobacco by adolescent males has reached as high as 43 percent in some age groups.[9] The use of smokeless tobacco by youth is generally higher in rural areas, in small communities, and in areas where there is a tradition of smokeless tobacco. However, high rates of use have been reported in large metropolitan areas as well.

To date, most attention has focused on the use of smokeless tobacco by white youths. Little information has been available on other ethnic groups, and some early research suggested minority youth were not taking up the practice. However, in some studies, Hispanic youth showed rates of use comparable to whites, and Native American rates were consistently higher. In most locales, use was less common among Asian and black youth.

Important for hospital-based health promotion programs for children is the finding that 60 percent of junior high school users and 40 percent of senior high school users believe there is little or no health risk associated with the regular use of smokeless tobacco. One-fourth believe that snuff does not contain nicotine.[9]

## Alcohol

In 1985, the percentage of high school seniors who had used alcohol in the past month was at its lowest since the High School Senior Drug Use Survey began in 1975. However, 66 percent still admitted to using alcohol. The percentage of daily users increased in 1985 to 5.0 percent, after having declined for the previous three years. Seniors who were daily users reached a peak of 6.9 percent in 1979 (see figure 9).[7]

| Year | Percent Who Used in Past Month | Percent Who Use Daily |
|------|-------------------------------|------------------------|
| 75 | 68 | 5.7 |
| 77 | 71 | 6.1 |
| 79 | 72 | 6.9 |
| 81 | 71 | 6.0 |
| 83 | 69 | 5.5 |
| 84 | 67 | 4.8 |
| 85 | 66 | 5.0 |

**Figure 9. Rates of Alcohol Use in High School Seniors**

The percentage of seniors who have used alcohol in the past year and those who have ever used alcohol has remained fairly steady from 1975 to 1985 (between 85 and 88 percent for the former; between 90 and 93 percent for the latter). The American Health Foundation reports that 19 percent of those between the ages of 14 and 17 may be problem drinkers, for a total of over 3 million young persons.

Abuse of alcohol (and marijuana as well) puts adolescents and young adults at risk of forming other addictions and dependencies and at risk of severe health consequences. The health consequences are diverse, but the association of alcohol (and marijuana) abuse with the high rates of motor vehicle fatalities in these age groups is probably the most serious. Data supporting this conclusion come from the National Highway Traffic Safety Administration:[10]

- Forty-three percent of all fatally injured drivers in 1984 were intoxicated at the time of the crash. This figure is down from 50 percent in 1980 and 46 percent in 1983.

- It is estimated that between 50 and 55 percent of all fatal auto accidents involve a drinking driver or a drinking pedestrian.
- An estimated 9,500 persons under age 25 were killed in alcohol-related auto accidents in 1984.
- Test results from 15 states showed that of fatally injured drivers aged 18 to 20, about 45 percent of the males and 30 percent of the females had blood alcohol contents of 0.10 percent or more. In the 15-to-17-year-old group, approximately 24 percent of males and 15 percent of females had blood alcohol contents of 0.10 percent or more.

The U.S. Office of Technology estimates that alcohol abuse may account for up to 15 percent of the nation's health care costs because alcoholics use significantly greater amounts of medical services than nonalcoholics.

## Drugs

As with smoking and alcohol use, the most reliable data about drug use among young people come from the National Institute on Drug Abuse's High School Senior Drug Use Survey, which involved more than 16,000 seniors.[7]

When asked if they had ever used selected drugs, 54 percent of the seniors indicated they had tried marijuana and/or hashish, 26 percent had used stimulants, 18 percent had used inhalants, and 17 percent had tried cocaine. When asked about drug use in the past month, 26 percent had tried marijuana and/or hashish, 7 percent stimulants, 7 percent cocaine, and 3 percent inhalants.

Almost 5 percent of the high school seniors reported using marijuana and/or hashish daily, down from a peak of 10.7 percent in 1978. Daily use for stimulants, inhalants, and cocaine were all reported at 0.4 percent. Stimulants appeared to be on a downward trend, whereas daily cocaine use doubled between 1984 and 1985.

## Seat Belts

A recent study entitled "An Evaluation of Child Passenger Safety: The Effectiveness and Benefits of Safety Seats,"[11] concluded the following:

- Child safety seats saved the lives of an estimated 158 children aged 4 or younger during 1984.
- Lap belts saved an additional 34 lives.
- Forty-six percent of child passengers aged 4 or younger were in a safety seat in 1984. An additional 14 percent used the lap belt only.
- Only 39 percent of child safety seats were used correctly in 1984.

- A correctly used safety seat reduces fatality risk by 71 percent and serious injury risk by 67 percent. But misuse can partially or completely nullify this effect.

Published in February 1986, this study by the National Highway Traffic Safety Administration points out that between 1978 and 1985 every state passed laws requiring safety seats for young child passengers. This seems to correspond with the effective use of child restraints in the 4-and-under age group. In 1984, safety seats and lap belts saved 26 percent (192 out of 743) of the fatalities that would have occurred to child passengers aged 4 and under. In addition, in 1984, 1,350 hospitalizations of children in this age group were prevented by safety seats and lap belts, and 231,000 children avoided incurring any injury at all as a result of wearing properly used restraints.

However, not all restraints are used properly. In 1984, only 39 percent of child seats were used correctly, up from 18 percent in 1979. This statistic makes the point that there is still a significant role for hospitals in educating parents with infants and children about the need for, and proper use of, child car seats.

It should also be noted that safety seat usage drops off sharply as children get older. According to 1984 nationwide observational and accident-reporting data, 68 percent of infants under age 1 were in safety seats, but only 17 percent of 4-year-olds were. A major factor in this sharp discrepancy probably is the fact that only 10 states require the use of safety seats for children aged 4 or older. Furthermore, passengers in the 10-to-24 age group were the least likely to wear seat belts.

## Immunizations

As a result of a major effort by the public and private sectors to encourage childhood immunizations, 97 or 98 percent of all children entering kindergarten today have been fully immunized—that is, they have been inoculated against measles, rubella, mumps, polio, diphtheria, tetanus, and pertussis (whooping cough). Percentages for children entering day care centers are somewhat lower.

However, it would be a mistake to allow the data to lull one into complacency about these childhood diseases. The 1984 rates of immunization among children under age 2 are much less satisfying, with immunization rates for mumps at 76.7 percent and rates for rubella (78.4) and measles (81.7) significantly below the national goal of 90 percent. Only the rate for diphtheria-pertussis-tetanus (DPT), at 85.8 percent, comes close to attaining the 90 percent target rate.[12]

Immunization rates vary by race and income, with rates for white preschoolers considerably higher than for nonwhite children, and rates for those above the poverty line or those living outside the central city higher than those living in poverty and in the central city.[13]

Reported incidences of several of these easily preventable childhood diseases also illustrate the fact that hospitals and other community agencies must continue to be diligent in encouraging early immunization. Incidence of measles shows an increase in 1984 to almost double the 1983 rate, after four years of decline. Preliminary rates for the first half of 1986 also were double the 1985 rates.[14] The incidence of pertussis increased in 1982 and again in 1983, followed by a slight drop in 1984 and another large increase in 1985. Reported cases of paralytic polio shot up in 1983 but are back down to just eight cases in 1984 and five in 1985. Declines in incidence for the remaining diseases continue to make good progress.[12]

## Working Mothers

According to the Bureau of Labor Statistics, there has been a "profound" change in the number of employed mothers, particularly those with infant children. In March 1985, 49.4 percent of married women with children less than a year old worked outside the home. This is up from 39 percent five years earlier, and more than double the rate in 1970.

The proportion of families headed by single mothers employed full time ranged from 38 percent for those with children under a year old, to 79 percent for those with children under 3 years old, to 84 percent for those whose youngest child was between 6 and 17 years old.

About 25 million children, over half of them with married parents, are in families where the mother is absent from the home for part of the workday on a regular basis, with baby sitters or day care centers providing care. Black mothers are much more likely to work than white mothers: 64 percent of black women with children under age 1 worked in 1985, compared to 49 percent of white women.[15] This may be related to the fact that the March 1985 unemployment rate for black fathers with preschool children was 10.2 percent, as compared to 5 percent for white fathers.

Working is necessary for many of these mothers. Two-thirds of the women who worked in 1983 were single, separated, widowed, divorced, or had husbands who earned less than $15,000 a year. Twenty-five percent of the women who worked in 1983 had husbands who earned less than $10,000 a year.[15]

Today, one child in five is growing up in a one-parent family, a proportion that will grow to one child in four by 1990. Forty-four percent of all black children live with only their mothers.[16]

## Conclusion

These and other data leave little doubt that there is considerable room for improvement in the lifestyles of today's youth. Children are starting to abuse drugs and take up harmful addictions at ever-earlier ages. Even with all the media attention paid to exercise, the physical fitness levels of school children haven't improved during the past decade. Problems related to weight are emerging as major diseases of adolescents in the 1980s.

Hospitals can ignore these growing problems and continue to treat the adult manifestations of youthful habits, or they can take an aggressive lead in preventing them. The opportunities are almost boundless, and many institutions already are making a difference in their communities. The following chapters are filled with examples of hospital programs that keep children healthy.

## References

1. Guthrie, H.A. *Introductory Nutrition.* St. Louis, MO: C.V. Mosby Co., 1983.

2. Children's Defense Fund. *A Children's Defense Budget.* Washington, DC: CDF, 1986.

3. Truswell, A.S., and Darnton-Hill, I. Food habits of adolescents. *Nutrition Review,* 1981 39:73-88.

4. Starfield, B., and Budetti, P.P. Child health status and risk factors. *Health Services Research,* 1985 Feb. 19:6.

5. Summary findings from national children and youth fitness study, PHS, ODPHP, USDHHS. *Journal of Physical Education, Recreation, and Dance,* Jan. 1985.

6. President's Council on Physical Fitness and Sports. *Youth Physical Fitness in 1985.* Washington, DC: The Council, 1985.

7. National Institute on Drug Abuse. *NIDA Capsules—High School Senior Drug Use: 1975-1985.* Washington, DC: Jan. 1986.

8. Hunter, S.M., and others. Longitudinal patterns of cigarette smoking and smokeless tobacco use in youth: The Bogalusa heart study. *American Journal of Public Health,* 1986 Feb. 76(2):193-95.

9. U.S. Department of Health and Human Services. *The Health Consequences of Using Smokeless Tobacco: A Report of the Surgeon General's Advisory Committee.* NIH Pub. No. 86-2874. Washington, DC: USDHHS, 1986.

10. National Highway Traffic Safety Administration. *Fatal Accident Reporting System 1984,* DOT HS 806 919. Washington, DC: Department of Transportation, Feb. 1986.

11. National Highway Traffic Safety Administration. *An Evaluation of Child Passenger Safety: The Effectiveness and Benefits of Safety Seats—*

*Summary.* DOT HS 806 889. Washington, DC: Department of Transportation, Feb. 1986.

12. U.S. Public Health Service. The 1990 health objectives for the nation: A midcourse review. Unpublished draft. Washington DC: USPHS, 1986.

13. National Center for Health Statistics. *Health—United States, 1982.* DHHS Pub. No. (PHS)83-1232. Washington, DC: Department of Health and Human Services, 1982.

14. Cases of measles in 1986 doubled. *The Washington Post,* 1986 Aug. 22.

15. U.S. Department of Labor. *Monthly Labor Review.* Washington, DC: Bureau of Labor Statistics, Feb. 1986.

16. Children's Defense Fund. *A Children's Defense Budget.* Washington, DC: CDF, 1986.

# Part II

# Designing Community Health Promotion Programs

# 4

# Creative Approaches to Keeping Children Healthy

Experiences of hospitals show vividly that those hospitals that have undertaken programming for children have been exceptionally creative and often aggressive in achieving their goals for these programs. They have designed offerings that are aimed at preventing the major causes of illness, injury, and death among children; that address emotional and mental health; that are fun and informative; that meet their health improvement objectives; and that achieve their marketing objectives related to children and their families.

This chapter discusses trends in content for community health promotion programs aimed at infants, children, and teens, along with some of the characteristics of the audiences they are seeking and the types of community groups they are cooperating with in offering classes. Case studies describing how two hospitals have approached the development and management of large community-based health promotion efforts for infants, children, and teens follow in chapters 5 and 6. Additional information on managing a health promotion series for children in the community is covered in chapter 9, Making Health Promotion Programs Work in Your Hospital.

## Program Content

In many ways, hospitals' community health promotion programming for children today is reminiscent of both their traditional offerings for and about children (hospital and presurgical orientations, babysitting, sibling preparation, parenting), and their wellness offerings for adults. But in recent years, many hospitals also have gone beyond these programs by adding new, relevant topics that aid both children and their parents in dealing with today's fast-paced and often confusing world. Programs focusing on handling crises (alcohol and drugs, suicide, kidnapping), on open communications, and on coping skills (coping with a divorce, with peer pressure, with working parents, with the death of a parent or sibling) are meeting the needs of today's youth. Community health promotion programs also are displaying their creativity and their responsiveness to children's needs by finding new ways to address traditional topics, such as by using so-called "well doll clinics" to introduce youngsters to the hospital and the basics of health care, and wellness day camps to help establish positive health habits at an early age. If current levels of activity are any indicator, the potential for hospitals' expanding their range of programming for their communities' youth is almost limitless.

## Audience

Although hospital-based programs for children are directed at all age groups, many hospitals suggest that children in the early and middle grades are most receptive to their offerings, especially during the summer months. Children of all ages—including infants—are being attracted to classes that stress parent-child interaction (exercises, infant stimulation) and communication. Several institutions also have found success in targeting specific groups, such as babysitters, youngsters who spend time alone because parents work, and scouting organizations. Medical Explorer Posts in hospitals are designed to encourage and promote health career development in high-school-age Boy Scouts. Other institutions work with both Boy and Girl Scouts to provide an extensive range of programming to help meet requirements for badges. Teachers, too, have been identified as a key audience because of their opportunities to improve children's health.

## Cooperative Efforts

Community health promotion programs for children offer many opportunities for working with community groups and agencies. Some of those with whom hospitals have forged cooperative relationships are the local Red Cross (babysitting and first aid), American Heart Association (CPR), American Lung Association (asthma, smoking), American Cancer Society (cancer education, smoking), police departments (preventing kidnapping, answering the door safely), fire departments (fire safety), park districts (bike safety), libraries (wellness programs linked to story readings), chambers of commerce (donations from member businesses), schools and universities (trained experts in various fields), Dairy Council (diet and nutrition), Tuberculosis Society (smoking), Planned Parenthood (childbirth education), the media (publicity), service groups (funding), and many more. Cooperative arrangements also range from simply using the resources of a group (materials, experts, volunteers) in hospital-sponsored classes to formulating complex agreements in which several groups work together to provide content, settings, audiences, funding, expert instructors, or promotion.

## Program Ideas

Following is a sampling of program ideas, ranging from the tried-and-true to the innovative, that are currently being used successfully in hospitals around the country.

### Tried-and-True Programs

Long before the terms *health promotion* and *wellness* entered hospitals' vocabularies in the late 1970s and early 1980s, institutions were already providing community health education classes for and about children. Most hospitals with a commitment to community education already had parenting classes—some quite extensive—and many offered hospital and presurgical orientations for children and their families. Babysitting programs, too, have been popular offerings for many years.

In recent years, though, hospitals have become more sophisticated in selecting topics for health promotion offerings, often using needs analyses and assessments of the health status of children to identify those topics most likely to improve children's health. Yet these tried-and-true offerings—orientations, babysitting, parenting and its more recent outgrowth, sibling preparation—continue to be among the most popular hospital offerings for and about children.

But tried-and-true programs need not be dull programs. Hospitals are finding inventive ways to add new zest to these old favorites.

### Orientation to the Hospital and Health Care

The primary purpose behind orientation offerings usually is to reduce the anxiety associated with hospitalization or emergency room visits. Having been introduced to the hospital's equipment and personnel in a neutral and even enjoyable setting, the child (it is hoped) will be less apprehensive if faced with the real thing at some future point. When conducted at the hospital, these orientations usually include tours of such areas as the pediatrics unit, an operating suite, and the emergency room; and demonstrations of procedures such as taking blood pressures, applying a cast, and giving a shot. And depending on the age of the audience, they may include actual hands-on experience in using a blood pressure cuff; stethoscope; surgical mask, gown, and cap; a syringe; and a nurse's cap.

Cabbage Patch dolls and the natural appeal of shopping malls inspired just two of the many innovative approaches hospitals are using to introduce children to hospitals and health care.

The mother of an 11-year-old girl stimulated the development of Marlborough (MA) Hospital's popular "Well Doll Clinic" when she observed to a health educator that her daughter was able to express her emotions and fears better than usual through her Cabbage Patch doll. Capitalizing on the popularity of these dolls, Marlborough Hospital set up its "Well Doll Clinic" as part of a city festival and invited girls and boys to bring their favorite doll or stuffed toy to be "immunized." Despite rain, some 500 children urged their dolls to be brave and learned a little about the importance of immunizations and good health care.

Following this success, subsequent clinics sponsored by Marlborough Hospital have attracted as many as 800 children during a three-day outdoor festival, and 200 to 300 attend regular clinics at the hospital. Each clinic is built around a theme, and each toy receives "treatment" in accordance with that theme. At the registration desk, each doll receives a name bracelet and an immunization card, and the waiting room includes a scale and equipment for taking height and weight, blood pressure and temperature, and so forth. In addition to all the publicity it brings the hospital, the "Well Doll Clinic" allows young children to encounter the health care system in a non-threatening manner and, by talking to health professionals about their doll's problems and fears, gives them an opportunity to express their own concerns in a healthy way.

A six-room mini-hospital, measuring 36 feet by 24 feet, affords Youngstown, OH, children "the hospital experience in a nutshell." In addition to showing youngsters the inside of various hospital rooms and departments, Tod Children's Hospital's "Tod Squad" characters greet the children, and staff offer casting demonstrations, show x-rays, and talk with them about health and illnesses. The mini-hospital is open at two shopping malls twice a year and attracts as many as 70,000 children over a two-day period.

*Presurgical Orientation*

These more specialized orientations vary in several respects, but they, too, are aimed at alleviating the stress and anxiety associated with the hospitalization of a child by familiarizing both the child and parents with the hospital, its staff, and its procedures. Most health professionals believe that children are likely to get well faster if their fears have been reduced.

Some hospitals conduct weekly orientations open to any child, regardless of the hospital to which he or she will be admitted. Others are held on an as-needed basis and may be tailored to the individual needs of each young patient. The latter usually are available only to children being admitted to the host hospital. Most are conducted without charge and show the child and family members the pediatric unit or area where they will stay, as well as the surgical suite and recovery room; acquaint them with specific procedures and equipment they may encounter; and introduce them to hospital personnel and routines.

## Babysitting

Almost without exception, institutions that offer babysitting classes find them among their most popular. At first glance, these classes might appear to have little direct bearing on children's health status. However, closer examination reveals that many aspects of child development, safety, nutrition, and emotional support are included in the programs for novice babysitters, many of whom will be future parents. Adolescents, usually ranging from ages 10 to 14, may learn about the following:

- Care of infants and children (feeding, bathing, diapering, formula and other food preparation)
- Entertainment for children of various ages
- Growth and development of infants and children
- General safety (often from the police department)
- Fire safety (from the fire department)
- Accident prevention and first aid
- Creation of a safe play environment
- Handling emergencies

In response to a growing number of child kidnappings, some hospitals include information on answering the telephone and door while alone with a baby or child. The "Tot Tending" class at Cottonwood Hospital (Murray, UT) teaches a segment on pet care, because many homes with small children also have animals.

But because babysitting courses are so successful, hospitals run the risk of becoming complacent and failing to find ways to make them better and more relevant. Instructors at Botsford General Hospital, Farmington Hills, MI, added a component on the business aspects of babysitting, giving attendees information about setting and collecting fees and operating in a professional manner. In addition, they set up a referral service so parents can call the hospital for names of individuals who have successfully completed the babysitting training program. The service also enables the hospital to gather names of the ultimate user of the class's information—parents of children being sat with—and offers the opportunity for Botsford to do an outcome evaluation of the class.

Community Hospital, Indianapolis, IN, includes information on the ethics and responsibilities of babysitting in its 12-hour "Super Sitters" class. Community Hospital also is starting two new courses for teens aged 14 to 16. "Senior Sitters" will teach the skills required to sit with the elderly who need companionship but not nursing care.

A second course for "Special Sitters" will teach teens to stay with children who have handicaps. All these courses have been developed by the hospital's director of nursing and pediatrics, and the basic "Safe Sitters" course has been packaged for sale to other hospitals, physicians, and professional groups.

Some institutions have uncovered a whole new audience for babysitting classes—grandparents. At Mercy and Memorial Hospitals (Benton Harbor and St. Joseph, MI, respectively), grandparents are invited to learn how ideas, equipment, and techniques have changed since they were parents. Classes cover everything from disposable diapers and infant car seats and preventing accidents to today's theories on growth and development and advances in formulas and feeding. The "Grandparents Discussion Group" at Magee-Womens Hospital in Pittsburgh includes current information on labor and delivery practices, infant capabilities, infant feeding, infant safety, and the role of grandparents in the family unit.

### Sibling Preparation and Sibling Touch

Another popular class readies youngsters, usually from 3 to 6 or 7 years old, for a new brother or sister. The classes may introduce youngsters to the habits of infants (they cry, they won't recognize you for several months, and so on), the basics of diapering (depending on their age), and may teach them how to play with tiny babies. Recognizing the obvious marketing value in these classes, many hospitals issue certificates of accomplishment to the attendees, provide them with buttons that say "I'm a Prepared Brother (or Sister)" and send them home in t-shirts with the name of the hospital and a message like "I'm a Big Sister (or Brother)."

Although probably closer to a patient education program than a community education offering, sibling touch programs (the opportunity for young children to visit and touch their new brother or sister in the hospital) are, for many hospitals, a logical extension of their well-received sibling preparation programs. But clearly, sibling touch requires careful groundwork and approval by both physicians and nurses. In most programs, young children are asked to wash carefully to prevent infection before being allowed to spend up to 30 minutes with the baby and one or both parents. Although health professionals were initially skeptical in some institutions, most have found no special problems are created and the family bonding that takes place greatly enhances the total birthing/maternity experience.

### Parenting

The child-oriented health education program that is perhaps most often offered by hospitals is parenting. Although such classes are not directed at children as an audience, they cover a diverse set of topics related to child care, birth, growth and development, and bonding; in all likelihood they were the impetus for many of the newer child- and family-related classes.

Today, many classes for parents go beyond the everyday issues of parenting and focus on situations that parents themselves must cope with, like "Step-Parenting" (Bay Hospital Medical Center, Chula Vista, CA), "Single Parenting" (Redlands [CA] Community Hospital), and "Expectant Adoptive Parents" (Botsford General Hospital, Farmington Hills, MI).

### Wellness/Lifestyle Programs

Beginning some time in the late 1970s, hospitals started experimenting with the terms *wellness* and *lifestyle* to describe health promotion programs designed for healthy people that encouraged and taught them how to live in a way that maintained or improved their health. Wellness topics most commonly addressed by hospitals included physical fitness and exercise, nutrition and weight loss, smoking cessation, stress management, and alcohol and drug awareness. Although these topics may have been a part of community health programming before the popularization of health promotion, hospitals, like other groups in their communities, began tying these activities together under the umbrella of wellness centers or community health promotion initiatives.

As might be expected, most wellness programs were geared to the needs of adults. But by the early and mid-1980s, a growing number of institutions were recognizing and responding to the need to keep children healthy by developing programs to meet their special physical and emotional needs. And today, as more and more families are participating in health-enhancing activities, the time is right for hospitals to aim wellness programs specifically at children.

It is estimated that as many as 40 percent of children ages 10 to 14 exhibit one or more risk factors for heart disease or stroke: overweight, elevated blood cholesterol, cigarette smoking, poor physical fitness, hypertension, and diabetes.[1] Although research has not shown clearly whether there is a direct connection between the childhood risk factors and adult diseases, the fact that heart disease and stroke are respectively the number one and number three causes of death in adulthood makes it seem prudent to prevent the onset of these risk factors by instilling healthy habits in children. In addition, the number one cause of death among children, accidents, can be affected immediately through prevention.

But one cannot take an adult lifestyle class and merely scale it down for children. Specific attention must be paid to the learning abilities of the target age group, their attention span, their physical capabilities, and their general interest in the topic. Following are just a few examples illustrating how some institutions have approached wellness topics for children through community health promotion programs.

*Exercise*

Children's exercise needs and capabilities change rapidly as they progress from infancy to childhood to adolescence, but even infants respond to physical stimulation. St. John Hospital, Leavenworth, KA, offers programs that teach new mothers to play with their babies in a way that stimulates the infant both physically and mentally. In Freehold (NJ) Area Hospital's "Wee Two" class, mothers and their 4-to-12-month-olds share their love and closeness while exercising during weekly fitness sessions. Gentle massage and stimulation promote bonding and social interaction while mothers experience stretching and toning exercises. Discussions led by health educators also cover growth and development, safety, illnesses, and feeding problems. An infant play evening at St. Jude Hospital and Rehabilitation Center, Fullerton, CA, reunites couples from the childbirth preparation classes for an evening, giving parents an opportunity to meet each other's new babies and to receive information about child growth and development.

Focusing on slightly older children, the physical therapy department at Grossmont Hospital in La Mesa, CA, teaches a free infant exercise class for children from infancy to 3 years and charges a small fee for a water safety class for infants through 4 years. Other hospitals offer water exercise for preschoolers and dancerobics for kids (North Country Hospital, Newport, VT), "kindercise" for 3-to-5-year-olds (Community Hospital, Indianapolis, IN), and aerobics for teens (Toledo Hospital, Toledo, OH). Toledo Hospital also involves the whole family in a "Family Shape-Up Class" that uses a follow-the-leader format to make it easy for everyone.

*Nutrition*

Parents today are increasingly aware of the importance of good nutrition for the entire family, but especially as a mechanism for giving their youngsters a head start on developing strong bodies and minds, and hospitals are capitalizing on this interest with special programs. Some are aimed at new parents; some are going directly to the kids, making good eating habits both fun and interesting.

Entitled "Baby Bites and Toddler Tidbits," Alexandria (VA) Hospital's class is designed to enable parents to give their children "the best nutritional start in life." Taught by a registered dietitian who is also a mother, it covers the nutritional needs of children from birth through 2 years, including breast and bottle feeding, homemade versus commercial baby foods, and mealtime psychology. Aimed at parents of slightly older children, Community Hospital's "Food for Tots" (Indianapolis, IN) addresses handling typical eating problems, discusses nutritious meals and snacks, and offers recipes and food tastings.

Children themselves are the audience for "Children's Story Hour and Super Snacks" and "A Funtastic Food Workshop." In the former program, sponsored by Bay Hospital Medical Center's Health Information Center, Chula Vista, CA, children participate in a story revolving around food and then make their own nutritious snack. The program involves children in the story through such activities as making headbands with antennae to get in the mood for a story about a hungry caterpillar. Then they might move on to making Easter baskets filled with popcorn, raisins, nuts and apples (instead of chocolates and jelly beans), or creating a nonfat yogurt treat with fruit, coconut and sunflower seeds. To help defray the cost, children are asked to pay 25¢ or 50¢ per session.

In "A Funtastic Food Workshop," the Nutritional Services Department at MedCenter One, Bismarck, ND, shows children in kindergarten through second grade and grades three through five that eating healthy can be "funtastic." The workshop is presented on various Saturdays throughout the year, and each of the two age groups spends two hours using games, films, and their own tastebuds to learn and experience the principles of nutrition. Among the handouts is a recipe book, *Sensible Snacks,* prepared by the Nutritional Services Department with graphics and recipe names geared to the children.

*Weight Control*

Weight control poses special problems for adolescents and teens because excess weight can affect a child's self-esteem. Attendees at a weight management camp conducted by Riverside Hospital, Kankakee, IL, requested a follow-up program because they felt they "didn't fit in" with their peers because of their size. Hospital-based weight management classes usually combine the teaching of behavioral change techniques with information about diet and nutrition and physical fitness. An increasing number of institutions also are involving parents in these classes. For example, Children's Specialized Hospital, Westfield and Mountainside, NJ, states in its brochure that parents are asked to attend the classes to help them "learn the best way to assist their youngsters in losing the desired amount of weight." Some institutions are offering weight management programs geared to an even younger audience, such as Carle Clinic, Urbana, IL, which has a program for children under 12, along with their parents.

Because weight control programs address an already existing health problem, it is not unusual for them to be taught by health professionals, such as psychologists, nutritionists, or exercise physiologists, rather than (or possibly in addition to) health educators. Some programs also originate in patient education departments rather than in the area of community health education.

More and more frequently, adolescents' and teens' desires to lose weight turn into dangerous illnesses such as anorexia nervosa and bulimia. Primary prevention of eating disorders is the goal of a session at Community Hospital, Indianapolis, IN, designed to teach young people and adults about the symptoms, causes, and treatment of these diseases. For those already affected, the Wellness Center of North County Hospital, Newport, VT, offers a self-help group that meets twice a month. Because the problem is becoming so widespread, hospitals also are beginning to offer in- and outpatient services to treat these illnesses. Linkages between these treatment programs and prevention activities can help alert communities to the problems associated with uncontrolled weight loss, including how to prevent it and what to do when the problems become serious.

### Stress Management
Although stress management programs for adults are extremely popular these days, surprisingly few hospitals have mustered their resources to design classes for children. Part of the reason probably is that relatively little research has been conducted about the effect of stress on children or adolescents, and even where research exists, not much of it has been applied to developing hospital-based programs. But the mounting teen suicide rate and drug and alcohol problems point to the conclusion that today's juveniles and teens are indeed under great stress. Hospitals are beginning to respond with a variety of programs that teach adolescents stress management techniques, address self-esteem, enhance communication skills with their parents and peers, and offer counseling. Crisis intervention programs, such as hotlines, represent an added level to stress management efforts. Because of a growing recognition that children and teens need help in dealing with the stresses of their daily lives, this area may represent one of hospitals' greatest opportunities for future programs for adolescents and teens.

A Family Life Series sponsored by Sheppard Pratt Hospital (Towson, MD) helps parents learn how stress affects their children, with such topics as "Teens under Pressure," "Communicating with Your Teen," "Drugs and Your Teen," and "Children and Stress." This psychiatric facility also recently developed a new audio tape service for use directly by children and teens. Called "For Kids' Sake," the program allows children and teens to anonymously call a well-publicized telephone number to hear medically approved tapes about loneliness, depression, parents' separation and divorce, alcoholic parents, falling in (and out of) love, and more. Each tape also includes suggested additional reading on each topic geared especially for young people.

### Alcohol and Drug Awareness

Although alcohol and drug misuse is a growing and serious problem with teens, a relatively small number of hospitals have developed programming. In those cases where the topic is being addressed, impetus, as well as instruction, often comes from mental health departments, pediatric departments, or school teachers.

One explanation for the dearth of community-based drug and alcohol awareness programs expressly for youth could be the perceived (or experienced) problem in getting the target audience to attend. But institutions have been successful in getting the message communicated by including information about drugs and alcohol in other related lifestyle classes dealing with nutrition, physical fitness, and stress management, by including it in sessions that discuss health problems such as high blood pressure, and by tying it to information on automobile accidents. Given the high rate of alcohol and drug abuse among the under-20 group, it is a topic that hospitals may choose to address more aggressively in the future.

### Wellness Day Camps

Rather than approach wellness topics one at a time, several hospitals have adopted a format that has already proven popular with many families—day camps. In these programs, children take part in a wide range of activities that are both physically and emotionally healthy. Three hospitals among those experimenting with the concept are trying different approaches.

A Girl Scout camp was the setting for a week-long wellness program at MedCenter One, Bismarck, ND. About 40 children who had just completed grades one through four paid $40 each to be taught that good health habits can be fun. Teachers included staff from the education department, the Wellness Center, and experts from other hospital departments. Lessons and activities during the week included a variety of exercises and games, fitness testing, fun with food (such as making nutritious snacks), daily swimming, lessons focusing on care for the back, "good touch-bad touch" (instruction in how to assert oneself when touched by someone, or in some way, the child considers unacceptable), first aid for children, and a family night. One of the goals of the day camp was to help youngsters feel good about themselves—a subjective, hard-to-measure goal, but one that staff felt was accomplished.

In Lebanon, NH, the Alice Peck Day Memorial Hospital decided to target its children's programming to the summer vacation time, and a one-day camp, "Young at Health," was planned. Forty-eight children, mostly in the 8-to-12 age range, attended the first camp, which was conducted as a pilot test. Children learned about smoking cessation, drug and alcohol misuse, nutrition, and fitness; tried new games; and engaged in healthy leisure activities. Beginning in 1987, "Young at Health" will be held during the mornings for a full week. The hospital received an award from the New Hampshire Parks and Recreation Department for its pilot effort, and staff responded well to the opportunity to work with children.

At G.N. Wilcox Memorial Hospital and Health Center, Kauai, HI, a needs assessment uncovered a large number of overweight children and those with high blood pressure, so a Health and Fitness Day Camp was developed to teach nutrition and other wellness topics to children.

Hospitals also hold camps for children with health problems such as hemophilia (Orthopaedic Hospital, Los Angeles, CA), speech and hearing problems (St. John Hospital, Leavenworth, KA), breathing/lung problems (Children's Specialized Hospital, Westfield and Mountainside, NJ), and weight problems (Riverside Medical Center, Kankakee, IL).

*Safety*

Programs on CPR, first aid (for both parents and children), introduction to the emergency room, safety belt usage, bicycle safety, poisoning prevention, and sports accidents prevention (often through sports medicine clinics) are just a few of the ways in which hospitals are teaching children about safety. Several interesting and enjoyable approaches to safety revolve around "events."

Every child likes to dress up, especially at Halloween, but costumes and trick-or-treating bring special hazards. So hospitals like Central Michigan Community Hospital, Mount Pleasant, MI, and St. Luke's Hospital, Davenport, IA, have used the October holiday as the setting around which to make children aware of basic safety principles, with emphasis on tips for safe and healthy trick-or-treating. By working with local libraries, St. Luke's reaches 900 children by distributing an easy-to-see Halloween safety bag and a sheet of safety tips to read at home.

Recognizing that today's children may spend some time alone or in the care of a grandparent or older sibling while parents work, the Children's Hospital of Philadelphia developed a basic first aid mini-course for children ages 7 through 12. Sponsored by the Emergency Medicine Department, the course covers how to handle fear in an emergency, basic first aid, what to do if an adult gets sick, and a tour of the emergency department. More than 200 children have signed up each time the course has been offered.

Through a cooperative effort with the city's recreation department, Alta View Hospital (Sandy, UT) provides information about bike, home, and personal safety to more than 600 children each summer. "Safety City" features a miniature city with buildings, including the hospital, and traffic signs (see chapter 5). North Country Hospital (Newport, VT), together with the Vermont State Police, sponsors a "Bicycle Safety Rodeo" that combines a bike safety inspection and a film on safety tips with fun and skills-building on an obstacle course.

## Responses to Emerging Social Trends and Problems

For many hospitals, showing children how to stay healthy is not enough; their commitment to improving the health of their communities goes beyond mere wellness. For this growing group of institutions, promoting health extends into the realm of problems and issues affecting society—and especially children—today. These problems and issues include adolescent depression, suicide, drug and alcohol misuse, child abuse, kidnapping, teen pregnancies, coping with divorce, communication problems, and more (see chapter 2, Nondisease Factors Affecting Children's Health and Safety).

### Dealing with Crises

Programs that help youth deal with crises are among many hospitals' most popular new offerings. Classes on teen depression and suicide are directed at a variety of audiences—parents, teachers, and adolescents and teens themselves—and are most often taught by mental health professionals or others with extensive training and experience related to the topic. Similarly, skilled professionals are most often called upon to discuss the problems of child abuse. "Good touch-bad touch" classes are reaching out to children with practical, easy-to-understand information.

Fingerprinting children has become a popular service for hospitals to provide as a method of helping discourage kidnapping. In some programs, police train hospital staff to actually do the fingerprinting. Tod Children's Hospital (Youngstown, OH) goes one step further by videotaping the children as well, giving the cassettes to the parents. More than 400 children, starting with the youngsters of employees, have taken advantage of the service.

Hotlines also are proving to be a popular way to meet social and emotional needs of children. In Los Angeles, selected teen volunteers are put through an intensive nine-week training course before they are allowed to staff the Teen Line, which has received 20,000 calls from all over the country since it started in 1981. Teen Line, open every night from 6 to 10 p.m., offers peers who will listen without criticism to problems that include suicide threats, drug abuse, and a full range of emotional problems. Cedars-Sinai Medical Center donates office space and a volunteer mental health professional supervises the four to five teens who staff the phones each evening. The program, developed by the Center for the Study of Young People in Groups, an affiliate of Cedars-Sinai Medical Center's department of psychiatry, was started with a grant from a private foundation; materials describing how others can start similar programs are available for purchase.

Cottonwood Hospital in Murray, UT, also has a hotline designed to help answer questions, allay the fears of, or provide assistance to "latch-key" children—those youngsters who are home alone until their parents return from work. Staffed by receptionists from the hospital's Women's Center who receive monthly inservice training, the Kid Line receives calls from children with genuine emergencies, children who are frightened, and children who are merely lonely or bored. The operators attempt to reassure the children as well as aid them in solving their own short-term problems—such as the youngster who was frightened by a noise in the basement. A discussion with a helpful operator helped the child figure out that the "intruder" was nothing more than the family cat.

The Kid Line also offers a Phone Pals service for children who are at home and feeling lonely. With their parent's permission, children volunteer to have their home telephone number given to a lonely child so he or she can have someone to talk with. Each volunteer Phone Pal lists a phone number for three months, and then can renew or drop out of the program. The response from both participants and parents has been very positive.

*Parent-Child Communication*

Programs emphasizing parent-child communication are being offered by several hospitals as a way of helping both parents and children become comfortable discussing the maturation process. In "Understanding Adolescent Adjustment Problems," pediatricians at St. Vincent Hospital and Medical Center (Portland, OR) help parents and children in their pre- and early teens discuss communication, social adjustment, physical changes, and how to work out problems together. "Growing Up Male" and "Growing Up Female" are presented by Planned Parenthood for Kaiser Permanente, Martinez, CA, as a result of requests from the HMO's own employees. The popular three-hour courses cover anatomy, social situations with boys and girls, and sexuality. Topics that may be sensitive, such as sexually transmitted diseases, methods of birth control, and making decisions about sex, are covered by the Magee-Womens Hospital (Pittsburgh, PA) in a class entitled "Mothers and Daughters: Making Sense out of Sex." A similar program addresses the same topics for mothers and sons. During a portion of the evening, parents and children discuss the topics in separate groups. "Morality and the Teenage Years," at Chula Vista's Bay Hospital Medical Center (CA), focuses on understanding the teenage lifestyle, including such topics as sexuality, birth control, cults, drugs, and the influence of television and music.

*Coping Skills*

Coping skills for children and teens is another popular category of programs, ranging from "Coping with Divorce" to "Dealing with Peer Pressure" to "Surviving with Working Parents."

Although parents and professionals are the audience, the objective of "Why Me?" (sponsored by Central Michigan Community Hospital, Mt. Pleasant, MI) is to help attendees recognize the effects of separation or divorce on children. At the same hospital, 25 7-to-13-year-olds spend a Saturday learning how to handle themselves alone before mom and dad return home from work, in "Surviving with Working Parents." Topics include fire safety, first aid, preparation of simple foods, nutrition, clothing choice, personal hygiene, bicycle safety, and pet care, as well as dealing with strangers, answering the door and the telephone safely, and dealing with feelings about being alone. The $5 fee includes lunch and snacks and, true to the point of the course, the program accommodates working parents by keeping the youngsters at the hospital until they can be picked up.

Many of the problems young persons experience in life can be traced to misunderstandings. To help children view problem situations objectively, explore them fully, and understand the ramifications of various solutions, the Gallahue Mental Health Center of Community Hospital, Indianapolis, IN, sponsors "Picture This," a group that promotes problem solving through role play. The improvisational troupe researches the special needs of each group for which it performs and then develops short plays dealing with such topics as sexual and physical abuse, death and dying, divorce, peer pressure, and alcohol and drug abuse. At a pivotal point in each play, the action is stopped so that the young audience can participate in exploring potential resolutions to the problems.

Even a health fair can be the vehicle for addressing social issues with children. One such fair, sponsored by Merced (CA) Medical Center, took on a new dimension because of the appearance of the "Kids on the Block," a nonprofit troupe featuring life-sized puppets depicting various disabilities. Illustrating the lifestyles of deaf, mentally retarded, and cerebral-palsied children, the "puppets" often find children more willing to talk with them than with "real" handicapped children, so they provide valuable information about being "different" while entertaining the audience.

# Reference

1. U.S. Department of Health, Education, and Welfare. *Healthy People: The Surgeon General's Report on Health Promotion and Disease Prevention.* DHEW Pub. No. (PHS)79-55071. Washington, DC: U.S. Government Printing Office, 1979.

# 5

# Case Study: Alta View Hospital, Sandy, Utah

## Setting and Environment

A 50-bed institution in Sandy, UT, just 15 miles south of Salt Lake City, Alta View Hospital is relatively new, having opened its doors on January 7, 1982. Its service community is growing rapidly (from a population of 3,300 in 1960 to 78,000 in 1985) because of migration from large cities nearby and because of a birthrate that is twice the national average: the average family in Sandy includes five children. The population is young, and over 50 percent is college educated.

The hospital operates a large emergency department, which existed as a freestanding emergency department three years before the hospital opened, and has departments of general surgery, internal medicine, obstetrics and gynecology, and sports medicine. It also has built a Short-Stay Surgical Center connected to the hospital. However, Alta View does not have a pediatrics unit; instead, it refers young patients needing specialized care to the pediatrics unit in its sister hospital in the Intermountain Health Care System, Cottonwood Hospital, in Murray, UT, 10 miles away. Two other hospitals also are located within a 15-mile radius.

Because of its location in the growing suburban community of Salt Lake City and the proximity of three other institutions, Alta View is in a highly competitive area. It has used service expansion, such as the Short-Stay Surgical Center and a clinic 30 miles away in the Snowbird ski area, to help gain a competitive edge. However, research conducted by the hospital showed that many nearby residents were not aware of all of the hospital's services. A decision was therefore made to use community health education as a major marketing strategy for drawing attention to the hospital, for giving parents and children a positive experience with the hospital, and for positioning it as the institution of choice for families in the area.

# Health Education Department

The responsibility for accomplishing this fell to Alta View's director of education, who holds a master's degree in health education and has a dual title and dual reporting responsibilities. In her role as assistant director for marketing for community health education, she reports to the hospital's director of marketing and public relations; as the director of education responsible for nursing education, patient and ancillary staff education, discharge planning, and social services, she reports to an assistant administrator. Both of these individuals report directly to the president. In addition to the director, the education department includes a community education coordinator, a secretary, a part-time coordinator for nursing education, a full-time coordinator for discharge planning/patient education/ancillary education, and four social workers under contract. This is quite a large department compared to four years ago, when there was just the director and a part-time discharge planner/patient educator.

## Children as a Target Market

Even more than in most communities, the focus on children in Sandy seems to be an obvious choice. Although children do not select hospitals, parents in an area with one of the highest birthrates in the nation are very likely to be favorably influenced by institutions that pay special attention to and meet the health care needs of their children. Thus the decision to use community health education programs, especially children's programming, as the basis for a major marketing effort was not only logical but responsive to an obvious need in the community.

## Programming

At the time the decision was made to expand the community health education offerings, just 7 programs were in existence. Today, some 50 classes are available each quarter, with 30 or more designed especially for children and offered during the summer quarter, and smaller numbers offered in the fall, winter, and spring quarters.

Although most programs are presented at and through the hospital, Alta View has experienced enormous success in working with the Boy Scouts and Girl Scouts and is just beginning to explore opportunities for working through the schools. After less than two years of expanded community health education efforts, more than 16,000 persons have taken part in the programming, 50 percent of them children. During that period, revenues increased seven-fold and the department was forced to go outside the hospital to find additional space to accommodate classes that ran a total of 10 hours a day, 6 days a week.

One of the keys to Alta View's programming success was its extensive needs analysis, sent to over 2,000 community residents, including children. It asked respondents to indicate their interests in some relatively traditional health promotion topics (babysitting, first aid, adolescent weight control, and adolescent aerobics) along with some unexpected and nontraditional programs, such as break dancing, karate, self-esteem, rocketry, and dealing with loss. A decision was made to attempt to provide programs for all top-ranking requests, regardless of their content.

Today, at any time during the year, children in Sandy are able to choose from a wide assortment of classes to enhance their physical and mental health, build their self-esteem, and improve their knowledge. Classes include "Teenage Dating," "Adolescent Behavior Modification for Weight Control," "Self-Defense—Karate," "Assertiveness for Teenagers," "Parents and Daughters—Maturation," "Parents and Sons—Maturation," "Babysitting," "Break Dancing," "The Dating Game," "Getting Along with Brothers and Sisters," "Building Your Self-Esteem for Youngsters," "Building Your Self-Esteem for Adolescents," and "Safety City."

In addition, a variety of classes are offered for Boy and Girl Scouts. Although the hospital had been offering such classes as CPR, first aid, and disaster preparedness, their content was not geared specifically to fulfilling merit badge requirements. With the help of local Girl and Boy Scout troops, classes were redesigned to follow scouting protocols. Now as many as 20 programs are offered specifically for scouts during the summer, designed to fulfill requirements for such diverse badges as personal health, dentistry, and fingerprinting. Classes are so popular that they justified the addition of another part-time staff person.

## Management

### Needs Assessment

Needs assessment has been a continuous process in Alta View's community health education area since an initial health promotion survey was administered at a health fair in 1983. Children became an integral part of the assessment process in 1984, when strong initial successes with programs for children led staff to seek further information from the target audience. An adolescent weight control class's participants and their parents were asked to take part in focus groups. Led by trained facilitators, the groups separated parents from children, asking each group what it thought of Alta View's offering an expanded summer program for children, what topics would be of interest, what were desired times and places, and so forth. The children, ages 8 to 15, were given small rewards for their participation in the focus groups.

On the basis of the focus group results, the hospital developed a a full-scale community survey covering four areas:

- Topics (in seven categories) of interest to children and adolescents
- Enrollment potential—the likelihood that children in the responder's family would attend classes at Alta View
- Media sources the responder's family looked to for information on summer classes
- Family demographics

The survey was tested on a babysitting class to establish its readability for children. The seven topic areas covered by the survey were safety, personal preparedness, science enrichment, death, adolescent issues, self-management skills, and "miscellaneous"—a category that included such classes as babysitting, drug abuse, and break dancing.

More than 2,000 surveys were administered. Four hundred were distributed at a health fair, with a 98 percent return rate. Another 1,200 were filled out by grade school and junior high students in health education classes. To accomplish this, a representative from the hospital personally met with health teachers in Sandy schools to explain that the proposed programs would supplement and enhance school classes, not duplicate them. A letter followed the meetings. As a result, 90 percent of the students who received the survey through their teachers filled them out, often during class. Another 800 surveys were sent home with students for their parents to fill out, and 50 percent were returned.

### Planning Process

Because Alta View is so small (50 beds), staff relies on an informal planning process that calls upon the skills and expertise of all individuals who actually teach classes. However, local pediatricians were involved in the development phase of the expanded programming for children through a special luncheon where plans for the summer program were presented and their input was solicited. As a result of just one meeting, a pediatrician who had not been a part of the earlier educational efforts asked for 500 copies of the program's promotional catalog to hand out during his preschool physicals.

Cooperation with community groups also is an important aspect of planning such programs as "Safety City." Initially, the hospital responded to requests for a general safety program by developing its own "city." But just before launching it, staff learned that the city recreation department was planning a similar program. Following a series of meetings, the two organizations joined forces, and more than 600 children received a much stronger program than either group could have offered on its own.

## Staffing

One of the biggest challenges facing Alta View in responding to the community survey was finding individuals to teach all the requested courses. Because the director of education has been with the hospital since it opened, she knew the staff, knew who was interested in teaching children, and knew which were good teachers. When qualified staff could not be found, she did not—does not—hesitate to go outside. "I look for the best-qualified teachers, wherever they are."

Outside instructors are identified through a variety of methods, ranging from word-of-mouth to official meetings to discuss the availability of teaching positions. Thus far, Alta View has never had to advertise for instructors. Instructors are carefully screened before hiring, and their teaching skills are evaluated. All who are selected are experts in their fields, and most have a baccalaureate degree as minimum preparation. The desire for and capability of working with children also are key factors in selection. Lesson plans are required and are reviewed by the director of education and/or the community education coordinator.

Instructors usually are paid on an hourly basis for their classes. In order to instill an ongoing commitment to the program on the part of the instructors, activities such as luncheons and an annual Christmas party, and occasional gifts such as flowers, are used to express the hospital's appreciation.

## Publicity and Promotion

The centerpiece of Alta View's promotional efforts is a 24- to 30-page quarterly entitled *Community Education Catalogue.* Copies are sent to a mailing list of 7,000 former participants and individuals who have asked to be placed on the mailing list, as well as the Sandy Chamber of Commerce, physicians, religious leaders, PTA presidents, and local libraries.

Individual flyers on selected classes also are prepared, and as many as 10,000 copies are distributed throughout the community, often through schools. To help facilitate this important dissemination mechanism, flyers are bundled into batches of 30, the average size of classes in Sandy schools. Pediatricians also play an important role in getting the message to children by referring patients, by handing out catalogs and flyers (especially during preschool physicals), and by keeping staff informed about emerging health education needs. At present, efforts to keep physicians informed about the program are informal, consisting largely of one-on-one discussions. Future plans call for a repeat of the highly successful luncheons for physicians.

In Sandy, churches are a key communication link with the community. A series of luncheons at the hospital for church women's auxiliary groups, during which the new, expanded program for children was discussed, generated a large number of attendees at the summer classes.

One of the unique promotional efforts in the start-up phase of the expanded community offering for children was the use of a billboard. Located on the freeway near the hospital, its simple message was "Alta View Hospital, Sandy, 572-2600—Community Education Program for Youth, June 4-August 24, 1984." The billboard space, purchased at a reduced rate, generated many favorable comments and phone calls for information.

During the first year of the expanded children's program, local newspapers—including those in Salt Lake City—were generous in their coverage of the programs, especially unusual offerings such as "Safety City," "Assertiveness Training for Adolescents," and the Scout programs. But programs aren't news forever, and Alta View is willing to place paid advertisements in newspapers to reach its audience and to keep the hospital's name in front of community residents. Radio and television public service spots also are a part of the publicity plan, and staff appeared on 20 radio and television talk shows discussing the summer programs for children.

As the program matures, so will the promotional strategy; everyone attending a community education program is asked where he or she learned about it. In this way, future publicity will home in on those media and distribution mechanisms that provide the biggest response.

### Fees and Budget

Although fees collected from programs for children cannot be separated from fees for other programs, the staff believes they account for a significant share of the $36,000 generated during 1984, a 700 percent revenue increase in less than two years. The department's goal is to cover all direct program costs, which include instructors' salaries, handouts, supplies, and textbooks.

The department operates under the beliefs that (1) all teachers should be paid, (2) all courses should carry a nominal fee, and (3) revenue will be generated by a high volume of attendees. Fees range from $5 for a 2-hour class to $60 for a 12-week weight control course. As an outgrowth of the high volume of attendees in all classes, an additional classroom must be rented outside the hospital to accommodate all the sessions.

### Evaluation

Attendees at all classes (except for very small children) are asked to fill out an evaluation form. This information is regularly tabulated and reviewed, and necessary modifications are made in the classes. But at Alta View, the major evaluation mechanism is demand for particular classes. Many of the initial summer classes were so popular that they were made available year-round. Fall, winter, and spring quarter offerings for children rose from 3 classes in 1984 to 16 classes per quarter in 1985.

## Benefits of the Programs

Even though Alta View Hospital has no pediatrics department, it has benefitted from its extensive health education program for children by making children comfortable with the hospital and trusting of its staff, and by convincing their parents that it cares about the health of Sandy's children. When a family in the area needs an emergency room, hospital staff—including the administrator—are convinced that they are much more likely to choose Alta View as the result of a positive experience one of their children had in a health education program.

The measurable results of the effectiveness of the community education programs are (1) a stable hospital census, (2) two classrooms used to maximum capacity, and (3) more than 16,000 attendees at classes, which is over 23 percent of the population of Sandy. The positive response to the community education program has changed the image of a new hospital from an unknown entity to a household word in the Salt Lake area.

## Advice

The director of Alta View's program offers five pieces of advice for those starting or expanding health promotion programs for children.

1. Find out what the community needs. This is the key to success with any audience. It takes a lot of time to do a good needs assessment, but in the long run it is worth all the effort.
2. Work closely with the pediatricians in your hospital. They have first-hand knowledge of children's health needs, and they are in an excellent position to promote programs and even refer patients to them. At Alta View, it was the pediatricians who first suggested developing programs to help children handle stress, and the resulting programs have proven to be very successful.
3. Hold the programs at a time when it is easy for children to attend. After school or on Saturdays are the best times, and summer is the most popular season.
4. Make the programs affordable. Set prices for children's programs as low as you can; the important thing is to get them involved in programs that will enhance their health. If the programs are good, volume will make up for the small fees.

5. Approach children differently than you approach adults. With adults, it is acceptable to schedule a three- or four-hour class. With children, think about that same class in modules of one hour a day, twice a week, for two weeks. And remember, they are likely to be tired after school, so their attention span may be even shorter than usual. Programs for children will take some extra planning, but it is all worth it when you see the results.

# 6

## Case Study: Dominican Santa Cruz Hospital, Santa Cruz, California

### Setting and Environment

The town of Santa Cruz and its surrounding counties comprise a population of some 200,000 persons to be served by this hospital, which is owned and operated by the Adrian Dominican Sisters. The only privately owned nonprofit hospital in the area, Dominican Hospital competes with two other institutions in the area, one a for-profit institution and the other a nonprofit, community-owned hospital. As an adjacent community to the burgeoning Silicon Valley, the Santa Cruz area attracts large numbers of young families who cannot afford the more expensive San Jose area, about 30 minutes away. The other major population group in the area is senior citizens. As with most hospitals in the mid and late 1980s, Dominican Hospital is faced with a declining census and is adopting a variety of measures to give it a competitive edge. Education is one of its key strategies.

The Dominican Sisters are a teaching order, so it is not surprising that health promotion was seen as being important. Although the hospital had several successful patient and community health education programs for children, they were scattered throughout the hospital. By bringing them together under one umbrella program, it was hoped that these efforts could help establish the hospital as a leader in health promotion and that satisfied parents also would consider using the hospital's pediatrics unit, emergency room, and child-birthing services.

### Health Education Department

When the Dominican Hospital administration made its top-level decision to expand the hospital's community health promotion offerings in 1983, it integrated into its programming a handful of health education classes being taught elsewhere in the hospital: CPR, first aid, babysitting, childbirth, and diabetes management. It was also decided to establish the expanded office within the Dominican Hospital Foundation, rather than keep the health education function within the hospital. As a separate nonprofit corporation, the foundation is the fundraising arm of the hospital system, but it also has a strong commitment to education. Placement within the foundation accomplished more than one objective: the foundation had the $20,000 needed to get the program started; as a small unit, the new department could move rapidly from providing a half-dozen programs to 50, and within less than two years to offer as many as 100 classes per quarter.

The Personal Enhancement Program (PEP), as it was named, has a staff of two, a part-time director and a full-time education coordinator. The former manages the PEP program, interviews and selects all teachers and classes, prepares the large quarterly catalog, handles the needs assessment and evaluation processes, and so forth. The coordinator manages the office, handles all aspects of registration and scheduling, does all bookkeeping, and performs a wide range of supportive tasks.

## Children as a Target Market

Through a formal needs assessment and interviews with the hospital staff, it was determined that the health education needs of the community, including its children, were not being met effectively, so Dominican Hospital stepped in, partly as a community outreach, but more important, as a manifestation of its teaching mission. Of the 25,000 persons the PEP program has reached in two years, it is estimated that from 10 to 15 percent are children. During summers, 25 to 30 percent of the class attendees are children. Although children were never a specifically targeted market, the hospital's emphasis on family care made children's programs a natural outgrowth of the expanded programming.

## Programming

When the Dominican administration decided that they would centralize all existing community health education programs and greatly expand their offerings, it was also decided that the PEP program would not be limited to narrowly defined health education topics, but would include a range of topics to stimulate both mental and physical health, to enhance knowledge useful for everyday living, and to improve self-esteem. Health, safety, and basic skills courses for children include "Alcoholism: The Family Disease" (one of three segments is entitled "Being a Kid in an Alcoholic Family"), babysitting workshops (ages 12 and up), junior aerobics (ages 8 to 12), basic first aid (ages 9 to 11), children's cookery (ages 8 to 11), gymnastics for tots (ages 2 to 3-1/2), and gymnastics (ages 4 to 10).

Enhancing self-esteem is an important outcome of such classes as "Color for Teens" (color and wardrobe planning, ages 12 to 16), "Makeup for Teens," and "A Day of Beauty for Teens." Parents are the target audience, but children are the topic in "Infant Massage and Bonding" (ages 3 to 6 weeks), "You and Me, Baby" (movement and flexibility for moms and babies ages 4 to 14 months), "Language Development" (ages 1 to 2 years), "Tempting Your Tot's Tastebuds" (ages 3 to 5), "Surviving the 'Terrible Twos'," and "Learning Disabilities—How to Help at Home."

## Management

### Needs Assessment

In the winter of 1983, a marketing firm was hired to gather information of use to the entire hospital about the health needs and wants of the area residents. Health education needs were just one segment of the survey, but some topics did surface. Although it was not necessarily as a direct result of the survey, the education department was established within a few months of its completion.

To get a better feel for the community's health promotion needs, staff also surveyed hospital employees. With information from both these surveys in hand and with some preliminary ideas for the PEP program in mind, a community advisory group was convened to help refine the hospital's role in community health promotion, to identify health education gaps it might meet, and to react to initial plans. Among the 15 members of the advisory group were teachers, a representative from the local chamber of commerce, a member of the local senior citizens council, a community relations representative from a local bank, several physicians, hospital representatives from departments such as pediatrics, orthopedics, and community relations, and others.

Needs assessment is a continuing process at Dominican Hospital. The 71,000 catalogs sent out each quarter ask for suggestions for additional classes, as do the evaluation forms for each class. New classes are added on the basis of these suggestions.

### Planning Process

Although the staff is small (less than two FTEs), the hospital is committed to presenting a wide range of classes (often totalling 100 per quarter) and so has devised a planning process that fosters creativity and variety and can be administered easily.

With the exception of a few "core" classes the hospital deems to be necessary (including babysitting, basic first aid for children,

children's cooking, and a program dealing with children alone in the home), all PEP classes are proposed by prospective teachers. Anyone wishing to teach a class develops a simple course outline and submits it to the program director. If the class is thought to be appropriate for consideration, the prospective teacher is interviewed, a resume is submitted, references are checked carefully, and a full outline of the class is developed. After evaluating the prospective courses, the public education director selects the courses and teachers to be offered in the next quarter.

In evaluating potential classes for children, the director looks for program outlines that are in keeping with the mission and philosophy of the Adrian Dominican Sisters and for topics believed to be of interest to area youngsters. Preference often is given to proposals from MDs, PhDs, or those with MPH degrees, because of the credibility they lend to the PEP program, and to experienced grade school teachers, to pediatric nurses, and to hospital employees who are known to have a commitment to the hospital.

## Staffing

As the previous section suggests, anyone in the community is eligible to become an instructor in the PEP program. From one-third to one-half of the classes are taught by hospital staff.

Probably one of the most interesting aspects of Dominican's program is the way in which its teachers are paid. Rather than receiving a straight fee, teachers get a percentage of the income from their classes. Under this system, no budget item is needed for instructors' fees; teachers are rewarded according to the popularity of their classes. In classes for adults, instructors are given 60 percent of the revenues generated. But because the hospital makes a big effort to keep fees for children's classes low, these teachers are given 70 percent of the revenue. Although this percentage is higher than many hospitals offer, it works out well for everyone at the Dominican Hospital because overhead costs are kept low and volume of classes and number of attendees is high.

All classes must have a minimum number of attendees in order to be held (often 10). A maximum number also is set by the director in consultation with the instructor, on the basis of the facility being used, the age of the target audience (the younger the audience, the smaller the maximum number), the number of instructors, and the type of presentation (for instance, lectures can accommodate more people than workshops). All classes are offered in the Education Center of the hospital complex, and it is not unusual for all six classrooms to be occupied by sessions.

## Publicity and Promotion

The PEP catalog goes to some 71,000 households in the county each quarter and serves as the main promotional vehicle for the classes.

It also serves as a promotional tool for other hospital services. In the Summer 1985 edition, "ads" were included (at no charge) for the hospital's chemical dependency service, women's diagnostic center, emergency room services, and family birthing center. Pictures of happy, healthy class "graduates," each wearing a PEP t-shirt, also brighten the catalog's pages.

A special "Open House and Registration Fair" is used as a point-of-purchase promotion. To encourage enrollees to register early and in person for classes, instructors are available to discuss their offerings at the open house, demonstrations are given, and refreshments are served. In-person registration also saves staff time in the long run because attendees fill out their own registration forms and pay their fees immediately. Students can register in two additional ways: Beginning the day after the open house and continuing for six more days, mail-in registration is available; for the six days following that (until classes begin), phone-in registrations are accepted. To make it as convenient as possible for students, Visa and MasterCard can be used to pay class fees.

### Fees and Budget

By operating "on a shoestring," PEP was able to pay back its $20,000 start-up grant from the Foundation during the first year and to generate an additional $20,000 profit in the second year (after all expenses, including salaries, rent, brochures, mailings, and so forth, were paid), surpassing budget goals. PEP's 1985 goal was to generate a $28,000 profit. This money goes to the foundation, but most of it makes its way back into the hospital to cover the costs of new equipment and services.

Dominican Santa Cruz Hospital has been successful at generating a profit for several reasons:

* Overhead is kept low through tight staffing (less than two FTEs).
* Revenue is maximized by paying instructors a percentage of the money they generate, rather than a specific fee (see "Staffing").
* A large number of classes on a wide range of topics appealing to a diverse audience are conducted. Children and parents are two of their key target populations, especially during the summer months.

Tuition for the "Teens and Kids" classes range from $6 for three 1¼-hour classes about dinosaurs to $22 for six weeks of gymnastics. Some classes also add a materials fee, up to $16 for four 1½-hour "Children's Cookery" sessions—but of course, they get to eat their creations!

A small amount of additional income is generated for the program by selling ads in the quarterly catalog when there is space. Recent advertisers have included a local department store and a delicatessen.

**Evaluation**

As is the case in most hospitals, Dominican Hospital relies heavily on forms filled out following class completion to elicit comments on both content and instructors. Because of the hospital's unique method of selecting classes and teachers, these forms become especially important in determining which classes should be repeated. To ensure that only those courses that meet high quality standards are repeated, the program director goes one step further. All programs for children are difficult to evaluate when the audience is very young, so rather than rely on attendance figures or unsolicited comments, the director periodically calls parents of preschoolers attending classes to ask how the youngsters reacted, whether they seemed to like the teacher, whether they appeared to have learned anything or have made the expected behavior changes, and, of course, what other classes they might be interested in having presented in the future. Because of this careful attention to both evaluation and needs assessment, Dominican Santa Cruz's PEP offerings continue to attract increasingly larger audiences.

## Benefits of the Programs

For Dominican Hospital, the mere provision of health promotion programming for children (and adults as well) is a benefit in and of itself, because it fulfills the institution's mission of providing high-quality education, which enhances the health and well-being of its community. Although this aspect of benefits hasn't been measured, with 71,000 catalogs in distribution, almost 25,000 residents already attending classes (although some are repeat attendees), and considerable publicity already generated, the hospital has gained a great deal of community recognition and support. In addition, the administration believes that recognition has contributed to the institution's good census. Staff and administration alike are convinced that when a local family needs to select an emergency room or other hospital service, it will remember Dominican Santa Cruz Hospital if it has had a good experience in one of its health promotion classes.

Through the PEP program, Dominican Hospital has firmly established itself as the community's leader in health education and personal enhancement.

## Advice

The director of Dominican's program has five suggestions for others attempting to create or expand their community health promotion programming.

1.  Plan carefully. Assess needs carefully, using a variety of techniques if necessary. Don't duplicate what others already are doing well. Find the gaps and fill them with high-quality programs.
2.  Wherever possible and practical, develop cooperative relationships with others in the community. It is good PR and it maximizes the hospital's resources.
3.  Evaluate. Counting attendees isn't enough. Take the extra steps necessary to determine which classes are working, which need improvement, and which should be dropped. Make sure the classes you offer deliver what you promise.
4.  Be innovative. Try new ideas. You won't make an impression in the community by offering the same classes that other hospitals and agencies do. Be creative in filling an identified need and you will be successful.
5.  Because children need a great deal of individual attention, limit classes to a ratio of 10 students to 1 teacher. If larger classes are offered, require additional teachers.

# Part III

# Designing Health Promotion Programs for Schools

# 7

# Schools as Markets for Health Promotion Programs

Children in schools, nurseries, and day care centers constitute an almost ideal audience for information, education, and behavior modification programs on wellness and other topics relevant to their young lives. By reaching children, adolescents, and teens in their formative years, there is the potential for encouraging and helping them to develop the kinds of health attitudes and habits that will ensure that they grow into adults with strong minds and bodies and for establishing lifestyles designed to keep them that way. In addition, both children and parents usually have confidence in the information that is presented through these settings, and youngsters are accustomed to being presented with new information there.

Unlike community programs, which seem to be developed most often as a result of some type of needs assessment, or based on suggestions from knowledgeable hospital staff, the impetus for school-based programs most often comes from the schools themselves, through teachers, nurses, or administrators. It is apparent that, in many communities, the hospital is viewed by teachers and school administrators as a reliable and credible source of information and education about a variety of health topics. Some institutions have chosen to go beyond responding to requests, however, and are aggressively pursuing relationships with schools to help improve the health of their community's children.

Schools also have been found to be a key conduit to the hard-to-reach segments of the community. Whereas it may be nearly impossible to attract Hispanic and Asian women, for example, into hospital-sponsored health promotion classes, they often are eager to attend school-based sessions that discuss important aspects of their children's health.

## Program Content

The vast majority of programs and services presented by hospitals in schools, or for schoolchildren at hospitals, address a relatively small range of topics—probably the same topics that were being offered before the advent of the fitness and wellness booms. They include various types of orientation programs (to the hospital, to the emergency room, and so forth) and health career programs, or they may fall under the catch-all category of speakers' bureaus through which hospitals attempt to respond to requests for presentations on specific topics by identifying a physician, nurse, or other staff person who can present a lecture or workshop.

Although programs for schoolchildren do not yet reflect the rich creativity that is evident among some hospitals' community efforts, there is a growing number of hospitals that provide a breadth of wellness activities through schools (including such topics as nutrition, smoking cessation, and stress management), that address the important issue of safety, and that have developed programs about current social issues and problems for school groups. The latter category sometimes poses special obstacles for hospitals because it includes some controversial issues and may require clearance or approval by the administration or others (see "Successful Strategies for Working with Schools").

Only a handful of hospitals offer school sessions that deal with chronic disease and long-term illness. Children's hospitals and those with active pediatric patient education departments have pioneered in presenting programs to sensitize both teachers and students to the special problems and needs of classmates with such serious and possibly life-threatening health problems as cancer, amputations, and diabetes. This area, along with programs addressing the social problems and emotional needs of children, appears to offer some of the most exciting possibilities for future programming.

However, this should not be interpreted as suggesting that health promotion activities are the only types of programming hospitals provide through schools. Indeed, other types probably are more common. For example, over the years, hospitals have conducted vision and hearing screenings in elementary and high schools and have provided physicals for athletic programs.

Initially viewed as community services, these programs were offered for little or no charge and were staffed mainly by off-duty hospital personnel. Recently, however, hospitals have shifted their approach. They now see schools as a segment of the community to which they can offer specific health services and programs; in addition to enhancing the health of students, such services and programs can also generate revenue or increase the use of other hospital services. Besides contracting with schools for those previously free services, some hospitals have expanded their athletics-related services to provide trainers, emergency services during athletic events, post-game or postevent check-ups, and injury prediction and prevention. Since some school systems have cut back on school nursing services, a few hospitals have contracted with schools to provide on-site pediatric nurses, much as they provide occupational nurses at work sites.

Thus, there is reason to expect that hospital-school cooperative efforts in both health promotion and health care services will increase dramatically in the coming years as more and more institutions look creatively at their options.

## Audience

Currently, most hospital programs focus on preschool and day care classes and the early grades (especially for orientation programs), with health career information being a frequent topic for high school classes. In order to expand their school audiences, some hospitals report working closely with health teachers in each school to identify those grades for which good health materials and programs are lacking. In this way, they meet specific needs and greatly improve the likelihood that their programs will be welcomed by the teachers. Some hospitals also target teachers and other staff as the audience for programs or topics, such as how best to help troubled students, how to spot signs of child abuse and do something about it, and, through sports medicine clinics, how to prevent sports injuries.

## Successful Strategies for Working with Schools

Many hospitals are eagerly sought out by schools to provide programs that complement their curricula or that fill the gap when the schools themselves have no formal health education program or, at best, a minimal offering. But others have doors slammed in their faces because health education in schools is not required by the state and is thus not viewed as important or appropriate by the administration or because someone within the school (such as a school nurse) sees the hospital's programs as a threat to his or her turf. In addition, many organizations besides hospitals are vying for schools' attention. Some voluntary agencies and service groups may be seen as more appealing providers than hospitals because they can provide complete health curricula, sometimes free or at a low cost.

Can these negative situations be turned around? The experiences of a large number of hospitals show that the answer is yes. Further, even when all the doors appear to have been opened because the schools made the initial approach, hospitals have found it important to continually build relationships with school staff and administration. There is a continuing need to seek out new avenues to meet the health education needs of schoolchildren and to help the school or school district meet its health education obligations.

Hospitals with experience in this area have identified a wide range of strategies for approaching and gaining cooperation from schools. Following are 15 such strategies.

*Survey teachers' needs and wants,* especially health teachers, related to health promotion for students. Programs developed in response to their requests are more likely to be accepted by them. Develop a mailing list of all health teachers and others in a position to provide relevant information and send a survey and cover letter explaining its importance. Ask the schools' central offices to insert questionnaires and cover letters in teachers' mailboxes. Work through the teachers' association to gain its support and cooperation.

*Meet with teachers and key school administrators one-on-one on a regular basis* to discuss how hospital health promotion programs can help them. Although at first this may sound like a time-consuming strategy, institutions that have done it attest to the value of the investment in establishing a one-to-one relationship with teachers who have decision-making roles related to health education/information.

*Work through school nurses.* Some hospitals have identified school nurses as a stumbling block to their efforts to work cooperatively with schools. Seeking their advice and collaboration, and finding ways to help them do their jobs more easily, can pay big dividends.

*Consider including counselors in the strategy.* School counselors may be in the best position to identify students' emotional needs and to suggest programs that can help them deal with social issues that affect their health, such as divorce, loneliness, and peer pressure.

*Identify a health liaison at each school* who will serve as the hospital's primary contact with that school and who will personally disseminate information from the hospital to appropriate teachers and administrators. Talk regularly with these individuals. Just before the fall term begins, consider inviting all the liaisons to a luncheon to describe the hospital's program and services and to identify additional ways to work with the schools.

*Meet with teachers, administrators, principals, and school nurses in groups*—either homogeneous or mixed groups—to discuss their health education needs and how the hospital might best serve as a resource. Somewhat less personalized than one-on-one meetings, this strategy still carries the strong message that the hospital cares about the needs of the school and is willing to work to develop a mutually beneficial relationship.

*Work through the school district or the health education department* to determine what role the hospital can play in keeping students mentally and physically healthy. Often it is most efficient to go a step beyond the individual school to the school district for approval and assistance in getting into the area schools. (Ideally, this step would be taken *in addition to* communications with local school staffs.) District offices and health education departments also may be willing to help develop a mechanism for surveying teachers, principals, and counselors, or to establish a process whereby hospitals can provide programs in all district schools.

*Implement these strategies with day care centers and nurseries,* as well as with elementary and high schools. Teachers in these settings have a wealth of information about the health promotion needs of preschoolers.

*Survey the children themselves through their classes.* Programs that appeal to the students, as well as meeting identified health needs, are more likely to be seen as valuable by schools. Hospitals that have built up good relationships with individual teachers find that many are willing to administer a hospital's needs assessment questionnaire to students during class time. Others will send questionnaires home for parents to fill out. Teachers in classes related to health may be willing to invite a hospital representative to lead a discussion about students' health concerns as part of a regular class session. Whatever the process, the views of students are critical to the success of any school health promotion activity.

*Select specific target grades or age groups for which limited resources seem to be available.* Experiences of hospitals show that teachers are often eager to locate education programs to reach groups of students for which they cannot easily find resources. For example, good materials and resources may be available for preschool and middle grades, but not for grades one through three. Or teachers may have excellent resources on physical fitness, nutrition, and smoking, but nothing on stress management for junior high students.

*Encourage satisfied teachers to tell others.* Word of mouth is often one of the best strategies for helping to build good working relationships between hospitals and schools.

*Work through the PTA or other parents' groups.* PTAs and other groups can have a strong influence if they recommend that hospital-sponsored programs be presented in schools. They also are a major source of funding for many school health promotion activities. Hospitals that are providing athletic-related programs and services have identified parent booster clubs as key purchasers of these services.

*Present controversial program topics first to administrators, teachers, and/or PTA leaders* to gain their endorsement. Topics such as "Good Touch-Bad Touch" for preschoolers, "Dealing with Alcoholic

Parents or Friends," or "Depression: How to Make it Go Away" may be seen initially as too controversial for presentation without some type of screening, and one or more of these groups may be willing to help.

*Send letters to all appropriate teachers at the beginning of each school year* to let them know what programs and services are available from the hospital. Early notification will give teachers an opportunity to work hospital programs into their year's schedule.

*Adopt a school.* Many communities have adopt-a-school programs through which local businesses offer a helping hand to schools in various ways. Through these programs, some hospitals offer student internships in the food service or printing departments. Some donate materials to the schools, such as out-of-date stationery or old magazines, which can be used to supplement school supplies. In others, individuals in the institution donate time to help bring a sense of the "real world" to classes in business, social studies, or health. Kaseman Presbyterian Hospital (Albuquerque, NM) has developed programs for both students and staff in its adopted school. Activities for students have included CPR training, career opportunities, leadership activities, poster contests, and break-dancing contests. Awards are given weekly for academic improvement, attendance, good behavior, and community service, and a monthly winner is treated to lunch with his or her parents, classroom teacher, and members of the hospital staff. Hospitals that have participated find the adopt-a-school concept gives them an inside track on developing good working relationships with the teachers and administrators.

## Program Ideas

The types of programs presented by hospitals for schools fall into roughly the same categories as do their programs aimed at the community: tried-and-true topics (orientations, career days, and so forth), wellness, safety, and (less commonly) programs that respond to current social problems and issues. Although not extensive, other types of offerings have elicited positive responses. Programs for schoolchildren on chronic disease and long-term illness and sessions for teachers, designed to better equip them to discuss and handle health-related topics, are just two examples.

### New Approaches to Tried-and-True Topics

#### Orientations

Just as orientation programs are one of the most widespread offerings for children through community programs, they also are one of the most often-seen activities for schools. Designed to familiarize children with the hospital and its procedures and to help allay fears should they ever be hospitalized, these programs usually are presented by volunteers or hospital staff who go to a nursery school, day care center, or school class. Using aids such as films, slides, and hospital equipment (stethoscopes, surgical masks, syringes, and so forth), the sessions are designed to help the children understand that the hospital is a friendly place set up to help people who are sick. Occasionally, schools will transport classes to the hospital for actual tours.

Some programs focus on a specific service used by children, such as the emergency room. Each fall, members of the day surgery staff at Freeman Hospital visit all the kindergartens in Joplin, MO, to show children what a nurse is and what she or he does and to discuss the kinds of situations that might bring a child to the hospital or day surgery unit. Joplin students through the third grade learn about accident prevention and what happens in the emergency room through "Accidents Do Happen." The course is presented in the spring because hospital staff have observed that there are more accidents and broken bones among children around that time of year.

A group of 12 trained volunteers at Abington (PA) Memorial Hospital will visit over 100 classrooms this year to introduce nursery school-children and first graders to "Poppy (Pediatric Orientation Program) Bear," who has recently been a patient at Abington. A slide-tape program developed by the hospital shows the children what Poppy did as a patient. His experience was such a positive one that Poppy decided he might want a career in health care, so he is taken on a tour of the hospital. Of course, the children go along via the slide-tape. A large, stuffed Poppy Bear accompanies the volunteers on each school visit, and the children get to handle some pieces of hospital equipment.

The national "Children and Hospitals Week," usually held in late March, offers a special occasion around which some hospitals construct events, including orientation programs. Sponsored by the Association for the Care of Children's Health, Washington, DC, "Children and Hospitals Week" is designed to increase the awareness of the public and health care professionals about the psychosocial needs of children and their families in health care settings. During the week, preschool and kindergarten classes are invited to make hour-long visits to displays at Community Hospital, Indianapolis, IN, in order to learn about the pediatrics unit, the kinds of tools and equipment used in a hospital, the use of seat belts and car seats, and the proper procedure for hand washing. The hand-washing display features a black light so children can actually see the germs left on their hands after they wash carelessly. The hospital uses a toy doctor's bag to introduce children to some of the tools and equipment used in a hospital, and then they get to see the real, life-size items. Attendees are given little favors (a key chain or a bank) and an apple. The hospital got so much publicity and good feedback after the first year's program that it didn't need to promote the second offering; schools called them.

Tod Children's Hospital reached 100,000 children in Youngstown, OH, during "Children and Hospitals Week" by sending educational packets to schools. These packets were designed to familiarize children with hospital terminology and specific programs at Tod Children's and to educate them about things to look for in a hospital. They included letters for parents, lesson plans and evaluation forms for the teachers, and activity- and story-starters for the children. Through questionnaires, children also were asked what they thought of the materials.

Mercy and Memorial Hospitals, Benton Harbor and St. Joseph, MI, have found puppets to be an excellent vehicle for educating children in kindergarten through fourth grades about hospital procedures and poison prevention safety. The hospitals have also used "Children and Hospitals Week" as the occasion to take their puppet show to area schools.

## Career Days

Several institutions have expanded the concept of career days to focus more extensively on high school students who have a particular interest in health or medicine as a career or who would benefit most from additional information about health and science topics.

High school seniors with an interest in health care have been taking advanced placement biology classes with the help of Abington (PA) Memorial Hospital and its physicians. Although many hospitals have difficulty finding health programs of interest to high school students, this program has been well accepted for 10 years. Doctors volunteer to lecture on a specific topic, relating the students' textbook information to what is actually happening in the medical field today. For example, a cardiologist and thoracic surgeon might discuss what medical scientists are doing with the heart, including current breakthroughs in preventing heart disease, diagnosing problems, and repairing the heart. A neurologist might discuss disorders of the central nervous system.

Similarly, Freehold (NJ) Area Hospital has targeted a program for gifted students in the intermediate and secondary school grades. The program initially was developed at the request of the Freehold Township School System to provide an expanded learning experience in various hospital departments and to allow students to work closely with identified staff members. The program has been expanded to all high schools in the area, following its initial success. Entitled "Health Experience for Youth" ("HEY"), the eight-week program offers an overview of selected departments, then each student selects four areas from the following to "experience": nursing, respiratory therapy, pharmacy, ultrasound, laboratory, physical/occupational/speech therapy, and cardiac stress laboratory.

Each student then spends at least eight hours in two of the selected areas, getting a crash course and learning to actually do one procedure, such as a urinalysis. In addition, each spends time in the Wellness Center becoming better versed in such topics as stress management for teens, death and dying, eating management, and decision-making. Participating students then put on a health fair at their school, teaching others some of what they have learned. A mini-version of the program is offered in the summer, during which time students are able to spend one week "working" in the hospital. Because many staff members are involved, schools are asked to make a significant donation to the hospital to cover some of the costs.

## Wellness and Lifestyle Programs

Although hospital-sponsored wellness programs are offered more frequently to community youth than to school students, examples of approaches to teaching wellness through hospital-school collaboration do exist.

### Nutrition

Visits by dietitians to schools are one way in which hospitals help elementary and high school students understand the basics of nutrition and begin building long-term good eating habits. Carson City (MI) Hospital has received permission from the American Dietetic Association to use ADA's "Nutribird" character as a special aid to help interest grade-schoolers in nutrition. The human-sized Nutribird presents the four food groups, discusses snacking, and involves students in planning healthy menus. In this rural community, several thousand kindergarten through sixth graders within a 25-mile radius of the hospital have been entertained and educated by Nutribird.

### Tobacco Use

Most hospitals that address the problem of smoking by children put their emphasis on prevention rather than cessation, even though a frighteningly high percentage of teenagers already smoke. The use of peer counseling as well as adult and teenage role models are two of the most-used methods to discourage students from starting smoking. St. Luke's Hospital in Davenport, IA, has capitalized on the popularity of the film "Ghostbusters" by entitling its two-hour smoking prevention program "Smokebusters." A fun approach is used to help fifth and sixth graders (and other grades upon request) grasp the dangers of smoking, to give them techniques to deal with peer pressure to smoke, and to make them aware that they have a choice between smoking and not smoking.

St. Joseph Hospital, Santa Monica, CA, identified a smoking-related problem for students, the use of chewing tobacco. Working with the local American Cancer Society, the hospital identified several premedical students who had an interest in talking to schools. The hospital served as a coordinator, and now local schools are able to add a unit on the dangers of chewing tobacco to their health curriculum.

*Stress Management*

As has been suggested earlier in this book, stress management programs for children have not been well developed by hospitals, either through community offerings or through schools. The growing number of classes aimed at helping children and teens deal with social problems and crises do, to some extent, cover the same content, but in a much more targeted manner. In today's climate, many schools are unwilling to approach subjects that deal with mental health, much as they were reluctant to take on sex education topics a decade ago. But a combination of factors, such as increasing numbers of students with emotional problems and cutbacks in staff counselors, has made both schools and students more receptive to basic stress management information.

Staff from the Mental Health Center and Health Education Department of Franciscan Medical Center (Rock Island, IL) have been especially active in offering stress management information through high schools in the form of both lectures and classes teaching relaxation techniques. Even first, second, and third graders are taught to cope with stress and pressures. By working through PTAs and other community groups, Franciscan staff help school-age youngsters recognize why they get nervous (a concept even first graders understand) and what happens to their bodies when they do. They are taught how to minimize these feeling through deep breathing, deep muscle relaxation, and other techniques. First through fifth graders also are coached in developing better interpersonal skills in order to help them deal with their feelings, understand the needs of others, and learn healthy decision making.

Through its Education Center, Sheppard Pratt Hospital, a psychiatric facility in Towson, MD, involves students as well as their teachers and parents in recognizing how stress can affect children and teens. A series of videotape vignettes presents everyday situations that can create stress for students—forgetting to get a permission slip signed by a parent, dealing with parents' double standards for two siblings, handling competition, being held responsible for a younger sibling while parents work, and so forth. Using a study guide, teachers engage students in discussions of each vignette and encourage them to suggest possible ways to handle the resulting stress. The same short films are used with teachers' and parents' groups to assist them in seeing situations from a child's perspective, in recognizing how they (parents and teachers) may be contributing to problems, and in understanding how seemingly simple circumstances can create serious distress for young people.

### Drug and Alcohol Awareness

An increasing number of hospitals are developing modules and programs to assist schools in communicating to students the dangers of drug and alcohol misuse. One of the most elaborate hospital offerings is from the Weller Center for Health Education of Easton (PA) Hospital. One of the center's four classrooms is devoted to drug abuse prevention education. Instructional programs are presented by health educators who are aided by sophisticated audiovisual aids and models, which depict how drugs affect various parts of the body. The drug education programs are designed to lend support to students who often feel pressured into using drugs. By providing solid factual information and examining the decision-making processes, students learn how and why to say no and still feel good about themselves. Alcohol, tobacco, and marijuana are the drugs that receive the greatest attention. The 4th- through 6th-grade program emphasizes how drugs can be helpful or harmful, depending on their use. The program for junior high students concentrates on the various ways people are influenced to use drugs. The high school program alerts students to signs of addictive behavior and suggests ways in which they can control their lives in a nondependent way. All programming stresses decision making, problem solving, and responsibility.

By working with local Kalamazoo, MI, school districts, Borgess Hospital and Medical Center has developed a series of health modules designed for grades 1 to 3 and grades 4 to 6, along with a teacher's workbook. In contrast to the Weller program where students go to the center, Borgess goes directly into the schools. In the fall, 4th- through 6th-graders learn about "Health Abusers—Drugs, Alcohol and Smoking." Prior to a visit by the hospital's "Health Factory," teachers involve students in a series of activities to help ensure that each one has a basic knowledge of the health subjects to be covered. Each module has a set of minimum performance objectives taken from material developed by the Michigan Department of Education. According to the hospital, the use of these performance objectives helps guarantee that all students in Michigan "will attain at least minimal competence to make wise decisions about their own health." Activity suggestions in the alcohol unit include an "Alcohol Facts Quiz" with true-false questions and an alcohol crossword puzzle.

The unit on drugs suggests that students keep a list of commercials and advertisements that promote a drug, identify why it is being sold, and determine what age group it is being aimed at. Another activity focuses on why people begin using drugs. During the actual visit from the "Health Factory," hospital staff set up hands-on modular units and show videotapes designed especially for each age group. Pre-tests and post-tests enable teachers and hospital staff to improve their program and help document the value of the visit.

### Safety

One of the most effective ways of attracting students—especially high school students—to a hospital-sponsored program is to work it into an already-established and popular activity. Kaseman Presbyterian Hospital in Albuquerque, NM, was able to integrate one of its safety programs with ongoing student programs at 10 local high schools. Its "Safe Ride" service is run by students already involved in school traffic safety projects, in an organization called Students Against Driving Drunk, or in a substance abuse program. Not only does it get across messages about safety and alcohol, it also provides a valuable community service.

### Sports and Fitness

Hospitals with sports medicine services have a variety of offerings for schools. The Center for Sports Medicine and Health Fitness of St. Francis Medical Center, Peoria, IL, has worked with schools since 1978. They offer a complete menu of services, including physical performance assessments, in-service institutes for parents and teachers, game and special event coverage, fitness screenings, and coaches' training. Each service is priced and handled as a separate product, though they often are bundled into a variety of contract configurations to suit the customer's needs.

Union Memorial Hospital, Baltimore, MD, offers physicals for students; coaches' clinics (a 2-evening course) covering injury assessment, taping, and emergency first aid; a 10-week class for coaches; and a speakers' bureau with 30 presentations for students, parents, teachers, and coaches. The speakers' bureau offers the first session free, with a fee charged for subsequent topics.

Parkside Sports Medicine Center, affiliated with Lutheran General Hospital, Park Ridge, IL, offers a portfolio of programs and services, including consultation for student athletic trainers, nutrition seminars such as "Eat To Win," and preseason screening evalutions to assess students' levels of fitness and predisposition to injury.

### Responses to Emerging Social Trends and Problems

One of the reasons more hospitals have not been aggressive in developing programs for schools responding to social trends and problems probably relates to the controversial nature of the topics and the fact that some school districts, administrators, and/or teachers still are reluctant to address these subjects in the context of health. But a growing number of institutions are successfully working through schools (see "Successful Strategies for Working with Schools," this chapter) to help students and teachers recognize and deal with the signs of depression and suicide in themselves and in others, to prevent child abuse, to cope with divorce and other family crises, and to understand the ramifications of teen pregnancy, marriage, and raising a family. Techniques used by hospitals for addressing these often delicate topics cover a wide range, including specially prepared videotapes and class discussion materials that aid teachers in making presentations (Samaritan Health Service, Phoenix, AZ, and Martin Luther King Jr. Hospital, Los Angeles, CA), lectures presented by hospital staff experts who involve children in learning new attitudes and skills, and experiential and simulated programming, such as involvement in high school family life classes (Carson City [MI] Hospital).

A unique approach to teaching high school students about the childbirth experience was developed by the Freehold (NJ) Area Hospital, with funding assistance from the March of Dimes. The purpose of the program is to give students a realistic view of all aspects of pregnancy and childbirth so they will recognize that, although childbirth is a wondrous experience, it should not be considered before the individual is mature enough to handle it. In the two- to three-hour program, a certified childbirth instructor lectures on labor and delivery, Cesarean birth, and natural and assisted childbirth. Films, discussions, and a tour of the labor and delivery unit and the nursery round out the first half of the presentation. Staff state that the actual experience of visiting these units helps the students distinguish fact from fiction about what happens when a baby is born.

The second half of the program consists of films and group discussions on adolescent pregnancy and fetal alcohol syndrome. Currently about 1,000 students a year are taking part in the program. Although initially developed for Freehold-area schools, additional funding from the March of Dimes has enabled the hospital to offer it throughout the state and to begin training hospitals in other districts to present the program themselves.

## Chronic Disease and Long-Term Illness Programs

A disturbingly large number of children suffer from traumatic, chronic, or other long-term illnesses and disabilities that make them "different" from their classmates. They may look different (loss of hair), act different (have a physical disability or abnormality), have special problems to attend to (shots or medications), or be absent frequently. Sometimes, both teachers and fellow students need assistance in understanding what is happening to their classmates and how best to handle what might otherwise be an awkward situation.

Orthopaedic Hospital, Los Angeles, CA, has found that all parties, including the young patients, generally respond well when the hospital's child life coordinator—along with the patients, if they choose—actually visits the classroom and discusses the situation with students. Prior to the visits, the disabled children prepare a series of posters about their illness, showing what they are and are not able to do, illustrating their likes and dislikes, and so forth. These posters are then used as the basis for the presentation and discussion with the class. Classmates usually welcome the information and the opportunity to openly ask questions about the illness without fear of embarrassing either themselves or their friend. Once they understand what is happening, they are much more sensitive and compassionate, according to the child life coordinator.

## Programs for Teachers

One audience sometimes overlooked by hospitals when planning programs for schools is the teachers. Health teachers appreciate updates and details about topics for which they may have only a superficial knowledge. Those not trained in health want assistance in how to handle students facing especially stressful situations that affect their school work. And the increasing numbers of suicides, child abuse cases, and children suffering from depression make all teachers aware of the potential they have to prevent disasters, if only they knew how. For example, Palisades General Hospital, Bergen, NJ, offers a program to help teachers increase their awareness of the problems of child abuse and neglect. "What's Wrong with This Child?" is designed to help them recognize symptoms of abuse and neglect, recognize child-parent interactions associated with abuse, and identify procedures for reporting suspected cases.

Although it is less dramatic than the aforementioned topics, many teachers identify safety as another area in which they feel inadequately prepared. Day care centers called Palisades General Hospital asking for safety-related programs with enough frequency that the hospital redesigned its CPR program to fit the needs of teachers of preschoolers. Through the four-hour "Baby Saver" program, participants obtain one-year certification from the American Heart Association.

In West Covinia, CA, a special program was designed for parents and teachers of preschoolers, aimed at reducing the number of preventable accidents to children in the community. Queen of the Valley Hospital developed the "Home Accident Prevention Project for

Young Children" ("HAPPY Children") with funding from their Hospital and Medical Staff Guild. As a side benefit, the program introduces parents and teachers to the hospital's trauma and emergency services.

The health promotion staff at Hadley Regional Medical Center, Hays, KS, saw a unique way to convey the importance of a personal wellness lifestyle to children by facilitating improved role-modeling by teachers. Working with the school district, the hospital modified its Aimwell health promotion program to meet criteria established by the district for in-service education. Consisting of assessments in physical fitness and lifestyle values, along with a blood analysis, the program was administered to teachers as a community service by the Medical Center and Fort Hays State University. The school district showed its commitment to the project by underwriting the direct costs of the blood tests. Over 75 percent of all educators in Hays have taken part in the project.

# 8

# Case Study: Freehold Area Hospital, Freehold, New Jersey

## Setting and Environment

Freehold Area Hospital is located in the western part of New Jersey's Monmouth County and serves about 100,000 people. The hospital has 257 beds, including 15 pediatric beds. Although there are other, larger hospitals in the county, none are close enough to Freehold to constitute direct competition. Built in 1971 because of a documented need in the area, the hospital initially focused on senior citizens as its main audience because of the many "adult communities" in the area. However, like so many other communities in recent years, Freehold has had an influx of younger families, and now both new parents and children have been added as target populations. In addition, as part of Freehold's transition from a predominantly agricultural area to a more residential setting, the number of schools in the hospital's service area has increased to about 100.

The hospital's administration and board are committed to the concept of wellness and continue to support wellness programs as "a dividend to the community" in return for community support of the hospital.

## Health Education Department

Freehold Area Hospital's Wellness Center was built in 1979 and occupies the entire west wing of the hospital. It serves some 30,000 persons each year through more than 100 different health education programs. The center's director reports to the hospital's vice-president for marketing and development, who in turn reports to the executive vice-president. Although the center has eight FTEs, only three staff persons actually work full time: the director, a secretary, and a marketing coordinator. Three staff members work half-time or more (a community health coordinator, a childbirth coordinator, and the mobile wellness van coordinator), two other clerical staff are part time, and the remaining positions are split among about 25 contract staff.

Wellness Center staff, who are responsible for all community and industrial education, offer programs in five areas: pediatric education, senior citizen education, childbirth education, general community education through the mobile wellness van, and worksite health promotion programs through the corporate wellness center. The pediatric coordinator, who is a registered nurse, spends a major portion of her time working with schools. The center's 29-foot van, a self-contained classroom, travels to fairs, exhibitions, runs, schools, and clubs. The nurse/driver takes blood pressures, offers vision screenings, and answers health-related questions.

### Children as a Target Market

The hospital's commitment to health education and the rapid growth in the number of young families in the area have made children a key target market for Freehold Area Hospital. Working under the philosophy that health education is a continuous process and cannot be achieved through one-shot programs, the hospital gears its efforts within area schools to reach all grade levels on a wide range of health and safety topics. Freehold Hospital's school programming is especially important to those schools in western Monmouth County that have expanded rapidly to accommodate the increase in young families. Parents in these families demand a lot from their schools, including health education. By working closely with schools, Freehold Hospital helps them meet the expectations of parents, at the same time achieving its own goals with respect to the youth market.

### Programming

Freehold's pediatrics coordinator has developed active working relationships with many of the 100-plus schools in the area, in some cases relying on a "health liaison" (often a nurse), who serves as the coordinator's primary contact with those schools. The liaison is also an effective and efficient communications link with other teachers and administrators.

In addition to direct verbal communication with individuals, each year the coordinator sends schools a list of topics that hospital staff can address. Topics include orientations and career day activities, programs on decision making and self-esteem, programs for gifted students, and classes on childbirth. To the extent possible, the hospital provides programs that meet the needs of both the students and the teachers. However, the hospital's offerings for nursery schools and kindergartens have become so popular that hospital staff now limit their visits to one program per semester per school.

Two of the center's staff members with backgrounds in social work and psychotherapy have worked with schools to develop a program that allows and encourages children to explore their own feelings and assists them in developing self-esteem and learning decision-making skills. Depending on the age of the students, a number of teaching techniques are used, including role-playing and question-and-answer sessions. Other topics covered in school programs include first aid, life-saving techniques for choking victims, seat-belt use, oral hygiene, stress management, nutrition, aging, death and dying, and smoking.

Two programs offered by the hospital have been described elsewhere in this book. One program, "Health Experience for Youth" ("HEY"), was developed as a joint effort between the hospital and the Freehold Township School System to offer gifted students a chance to spend eight days in the hospital working with specially selected staff members in various departments (see chapter 7 under "New Approaches to Tried-and-True Topics").

The second program, "Orientation to Childbirth for High School Students," provides students with accurate, factual information about childbirth so they can make well-founded decisions about becoming parents. According to Wellness Center staff, the program is not seen as controversial by the community because it does not make judgments about what is or is not "right." Rather, it gives the students information and a framework for decision-making so they can decide for themselves what is right. (See chapter 7 under "Responses to Emerging Social Trends and Problems.")

Before the hospital visit, classroom teachers give students a test that asks a few basic questions about childbirth, such as the average length of labor for a first-time mother, and the effects of a mother's eating, drinking, and smoking habits on her unborn child. The results of these tests are used by the childbirth education coordinator to tailor each presentation to meet the needs of the specific class. A post-visit test provides feedback on what was learned. After five years, the course continues to attract 1,000 high school students yearly and is a valued component of many health, family life, physical education, and home economics curricula.

## Management

### Needs Assessment

With some exceptions, programs are developed by the Wellness Center on the basis of a needs assessment. For some classes, the need is well established and the center merely responds with appropriate programming. The need for programs on breast self-examination, even for adolescents, is one example. For other topics, requests from knowledgeable staff or from schools are enough to stimulate the development of a course.

For most programs, however, development is preceded by some kind of needs analysis. For instance, before the "Family Asthma Program" was developed, an extensive assessment was done by contacting between 50 and 60 school nurses and others to learn not only whether they thought it was necessary, but also where and when it should be held, what aspects of the topic should be covered, and so forth. Staff also caution that even when a needs assessment *does* show that a class is "needed," that finding does not guarantee that people will attend. Although poorly attended classes are discontinued, staff are encouraged to learn from those experiences and use them to improve future offerings.

## Planning Process

The Wellness Center's four coordinators meet twice a month. When a new class is suggested, a coordinator is assigned to research the topic, do a needs analysis for that topic, and involve the appropriate additional staff in developing the curriculum. In the case of programs for schools, it is usual for school nurses, teachers, or principals to be involved in planning. After a course has been developed, it is presented to the Medical Advisory Committee of the Wellness Center. The committee, which meets quarterly, must approve all new offerings.

## Staffing

Although the pediatrics coordinator teaches the core program offerings in schools, others on the Wellness Center staff also may be involved as needed to bring expertise to a particular topic. To supplement the staff, the center has 25 instructors under contract to teach programs for children. Programs can therefore be delivered by a number of individuals. For instance, the childbirth coordinator teaches the "Orientation to Childbirth" classes, a nutritionist presents a diet class for teens, and a psychotherapist teaches the decision-making section in the "HEY" program.

## Publicity and Promotion

Five coordinated brochures, each describing one of the five divisions within Freehold Area Hospital's Wellness Center, are issued semi-annually. These brochures serve as the major source of publicity and promotion for the center's programs. A recently hired marketing coordinator now handles these brochures and all promotional activities of the center. Press releases highlighting special or unusual programs are sent to 20 newspapers covering the hospital's service area. Notices in PTA bulletins have proven to be effective in promoting activities in schools. Occasionally the center places paid ads; however, because most programs for schools are offered free of charge, there seldom is revenue to cover the cost of paid ads for these offerings.

The hospital's strong relationships with many schools pay off when it comes to promoting their programming: some teachers send brochures on the pediatric education offerings home with students. Some schools even go so far as to reproduce Freehold's materials for distribution to the children, while others will disseminate material but require prior approval of the content before they do so.

## Fees and Budget

Because of the hospital's strong commitment to providing health promotion programming for children, most of the pediatric education offerings are subsidized by the institution. Therefore, although the overall goal of the Wellness Center is to break even, only a few school classes—like the "HEY" program for gifted children—require any kind of fee or donation. Others, such as the "Orientation to Childbirth" program, were originally developed under a grant but will be continued as a service of the institution. If, however, a school requests a special program that requires a great deal of staff time to develop, or if an individual school requests a large number of classes, the center charges a small fee. In order to enable schools to budget for fees where necessary, most special programs are scheduled up to a year in advance. Fees vary depending on the amount of staff time required to develop and present the programs, as well as the direct costs involved.

Instructors in classes for children are reimbursed in one of three ways. Teachers employed by the Wellness Center present programs for children as part of their jobs, so their regular salary covers all their time. Staff members from other departments in the hospital who teach programs for children are paid an hourly rate for their teaching time. As a small added incentive, Freehold pays staff for 15 minutes before and after the actual class time. Finally, contract instructors are paid on an hourly basis for the classes they teach.

## Evaluation

Whenever possible, tests relating to the subject to be covered are developed by the hospital and administered to students by their teachers before and after presentations. Information from these tests, combined with feedback from classroom teachers themselves, provides the primary source of evaluation information for Freehold's school programs. But some classes, such as the "HEY" and "Orientation to Childbirth" programs, also require evaluation sheets to be filled out by students. The questionnaire following the "HEY" program asks why the student chose the program, what was most interesting about the program, what was most helpful, what was least interesting and least helpful, whether the class met the student's expectations, whether he or she would attend again or recommend it to a friend, and so forth.

Except for feedback from classroom teachers, programs for very young students usually are not formally evaluated.

## Benefits of the Programs

To Freehold Area Hospital, the major benefit of presenting health promotion programs to children through schools is the opportunity to develop good health care consumers and healthy community residents by encouraging children and teens to adopt good health habits early. Their wellness activities give the hospital the ability to "care for" the well in their community in addition to the sick. Improved community relations and good public relations are a bonus.

## Advice

The director of Freehold Area Hospital's Wellness Center offers four pieces of advice to others working with schools:

1. Find out what your hospital can do best to help local schools and stick to that. School teachers know how to do a lot. They frequently (and adeptly) manage many activities at once and usually are very well organized and well qualified. Try to find the gaps and fill them. Do for them what they cannot do for themselves.

2. Within those "gaps," be creative. Be willing to try anything. New ideas may not all work, but as long as staff members learn from their experience and improve future offerings, the process probably will have been worthwhile. And when innovative ideas do produce good, popular programs, everyone, including the staff, will get a big boost.

3. When developing programs with an individual school, share resources to the extent possible so that everyone involved "owns" a piece of the final product. If the school makes a contribution to the program in the form of a fee, planning time, or materials, it will have a stronger commitment to the program's success.

4. When selecting teachers for programs aimed at children, look for individuals who have experience working with children, a health *education* background, and a strong general health background in addition to their areas of special expertise. A well-rounded background in a variety of health topics is important because students often ask questions on a wide range of topics that are frequently far removed from the immediate subject of the class.

# Part IV

# Managing Health Promotion Programs for Children and Youth

# 9

# Making Health Promotion Programs Work in Your Hospital

When planning health promotion programs for children, regardless of whether they are programs for the community or for schools, it is easy to fall into the trap of thinking only about program *content* and forgetting about the all-important area of program *management*. It is true that in most hospitals, with the possible exception of children's hospitals, the management of health promotion programs for children is not separated from programs designed for other audiences. But although there may be little difference in some management aspects—the departments in which these programs originate, for example—there is considerable difference in other aspects, such as how needs assessments and evaluations are conducted, especially for very young children.

Following is an examination of some management issues that should be considered when a hospital contemplates undertaking, expanding, or reassessing its health promotion programming for and about children. Also included are examples of how specific hospitals have approached the issues. The list of management topics is not meant to be exhaustive, nor are the approaches reported meant to represent the "best" practices, since in most areas no one approach can be said to be the "best" for all institutions. Rather, they are presented to assist the reader in planning future programs and to stimulate the development of creative and innovative responses to ever-present situations and problems. (The case studies presented in chapters 5, 6, and 8 give detailed illustrations of many aspects of program management.)

## Organizational Structure

Differences in organizational structure of children's programs within a hospital may reflect differences in program focus. Many health promotion programs for and about children originate in the hospital department that is responsible for other community health education programs. For institutions in which community health education is the primary or sole focus of the department, it may be called health promotion, community health education, health information, or family health, or it may be part of a wellness center. But it also is common for childrens' health promotion activities to be centered in departments with multiple responsibilities, including nursing education, patient education, staff education, and so forth. In some institutions, childrens' programs are located in more than one department.

The most common pattern the authors found in gathering information for this book is for hospitals to separate programs that deal with lifestyles of healthy children (physical fitness, nutrition, coping skills) from those that help youngsters with health problems (weight reduction classes, breathing camps) or those that are related to medical procedures (sibling visit programs following the birth of a brother or sister, presurgical orientations). In hospitals following this pattern, the lifestyle programs might be located in the community health education department, while health-problem and medical-procedure programs might be found in the nursing or patient education department.

Programs that are targeted to schools generally follow the same pattern—that is, lifestyle programs originate in a community-focused department, while programs addressing health or medical problems may come from a more specialized department. School programs also may originate in volunteer or auxiliary departments.

Although it is far from a hard-and-fast rule, the most common pattern for sponsoring departments is for their directors to report to a vice-president who in turn reports to the hospital's CEO or administrator. In general, community and school health education programs are directed by middle management personnel, who appear to have access to top decision-makers. If one or more individuals have specific responsibility for childrens' health promotion programming, they usually report to the director of the sponsoring or originating department.

## Personnel

### Size of Staff

Because programs for children usually are just one function in a larger department, there is almost no correlation between the size of the department and the size of the program staff. Some hospitals offering dozens of programs for children each summer have only one or two full-time staff members, whereas many hospitals with large health education staffs offer only a few classes for youngsters. Therefore, it is not possible to generalize about the number of staff hospitals have found necessary to successfully run programs for children.

## Sources of Staff

Some staffing patterns emerge when one looks at the types of personnel most often involved with programs for children. Certainly, health educators are the staff most often used for both planning and teaching programs. But as might be expected, nurses, especially pediatric nurses, are heavily involved in teaching children. They are likely to have advanced degrees in education, work experience in education or counseling, or a strong interest in working with children. Some program directors state that they always look for teachers who have a strong interest in children or who are themselves parents.

Others who might make suitable teachers for children are hospital staff—some because of their medical expertise, such as nutritionists or physical therapists; some because of their administrative background, such as admitting clerks who provide presurgical orientations to children or give instruction on using infant car seats to registering maternity patients. Volunteers and auxilians also are called on as teachers, especially for school programs.

Preferences vary as to how heavily hospitals rely on their own staff as teachers. A director of health education in a North Dakota hospital said she would "get static" if she went outside the hospital for teachers, and Community Hospital in Indianapolis, IN, uses 90 percent in-house staff. But other hospitals rely heavily on instructors from the community or give no preference to their staff.

Similar criteria are used in selecting teachers from the community as in selecting them from within the hospital—experience with and an interest in children, or the experience of being a parent who has "been through it." Tod Children's Hospital, Youngstown, OH, finds that "Foster Grandparents" fit these criteria and are excellent with children, including inpatients. The "Grandparents" are given specific assignments each day and are paid for their work.

## Compensation

Compensation practices also differ among hospitals. At St. Luke's Hospital, Davenport, IA, and St. Jude Hospital, Fullerton, CA, inpatient teaching is part of the professional nurse's job description, so staff are not given compensatory time for special education program commitments. At the other end of the scale, staff teachers at Central Michigan Community Hospital, Mount Pleasant, MI, are paid additional compensation beyond their salaries for any responsibilities added to their jobs. At some institutions, a middle line is taken: staff are paid or given compensatory time if a program requires them to work overtime.

Although some hospitals still call on volunteers from the community to teach health promotion classes, a growing number prefer to hire nonhospital teachers on contract. The most common reason given for preferring to pay teachers is to ensure greater control over the content and quality of programs. Most contract arrangements specify a fee for teaching a certain number of classes or a predetermined number of hours, but some hospitals have come up with innovative arrangements, such as Dominican Santa Cruz (CA) Hospital, which gives community teachers a percentage of the fees generated by their course. This arrangement not only eliminates a budget line for teachers' fees, but it also rewards instructors according to the success of their programs. Hospitals may also contract with teachers on a monthly basis to cover specific teaching responsibilities and additional services (developing materials or assisting with office duties such as class registration).

### Training

Many hospitals that offer programming for children seek out instructors who have a good track record in working with children, often elementary school teachers, pediatric nurses, or qualified parents. Although individuals in the latter two categories may have excellent skills for dealing with children, they often lack actual classroom teaching experience. Many hospital staff members, too, are eager to work with children but have never conducted a class.

To help overcome any shortcomings in teaching skills, some institutions offer special training sessions covering such topics as the philosophy of and services offered by the hospital, principles of education, stages of child development (focusing on the differing needs of various age groups), teaching methods, and so forth. Those hospitals equipped with videotape capabilities may even offer teachers the opportunity to view and critique their own classroom performance. Where a training program is not practical, hospitals can give each teacher an orientation packet. Whatever the vehicle, all instructors new to a program should receive information about what is expected in terms of reports (attendance records, evaluations, and so forth) and how to handle emergencies.

## Planning

The degree of formality involved in planning children's health promotion programs is often a function of the relationship between the sponsoring department (community health education, nursing, or whatever) and the rest of the hospital. The size of the hospital may also be a factor, with large ones undertaking a more formal planning process than small ones.

## Internal Planning Arrangements

For institutions in which a formal planning mechanism is needed, a variety of models can be used. One of the most common models brings together staff or department heads from the involved areas so that each can contribute to the design of a new program (MedCenter One, Bismarck, ND). A similar but less far-reaching technique calls for a health educator to serve as an educational consultant to the hospital staff from other departments who will actually teach the classes (Bay City Medical Center, Chula Vista, CA).

Sometimes specific committees are designated as part of the planning process; these committees often include physicans. At Freehold (NJ) Area Hospital, topics are assigned to an education coordinator, who researches the topic and involves appropriate staff experts in planning the content. The program is then taken to the Medical Advisory Committee of the Wellness Center, which meets quarterly and must approve all the center's programs.

## Planning with Community Groups

As more and more hospitals involve community groups and agencies in their health promotion programs for children, attention must be given to how groups will work together, how expenses will be handled, how cooperating groups will be credited in promotional material, which group will control the content and promotion of the program, which will handle logistics, and so forth (see also Use of Community Groups, below).

By approaching community groups with already-established activities for children, St. Luke's Hospital, Davenport, IA, was able to maintain complete control of the health promotion content of its "Halloween Safety Program" (done through the library) and its "Summer Playground Program" (done with the park system). By contrast, a great deal of cooperative planning and negotiation may be necessary to avoid duplication of efforts, as was the case when Alta View Hospital (Sandy, UT) and the local park district found they had planned similar and overlapping "Safety City" programs.

## Planning School-Based Programs

Hospitals' experiences vary regarding the amount of joint planning required when working with schools. Although it is not recommended, the most common approach seems to be for hospitals to plan programs without direct involvement by the school system. Some hospitals do involve school health nurses, selected teachers, and administrators in the needs analysis; others, like Kaweah District Hospital, Visalia, CA, work closely with school nurses or the school health education department to ensure that programs taken into the school mesh with the school health education curriculum.

Borgess Medical Center, Kalamazoo, MI, worked extensively with teachers to develop a series of health modules and a teaching workbook. Now teachers register in advance and agree to use the workbook before "Borgee's (a mascot) Health Factory" visits the school. Hospitals also have gotten good results from involving students themselves in the planning process (see Needs Assessment: Children's Involvement, below).

In developing cooperative programs with schools or with any outside group, it is vital that hospital representatives be well briefed before entering discussions about what the hospital can and cannot offer. Discussions will be most effective when all promises can be kept and when the individual involved in the negotiations has the authority to make decisions and commitments.

## Use of Community Groups

### Types of Groups Available

Hospitals are using a rich assortment of community groups in implementing their health promotion programs for children. In addition to such well-known voluntary agencies as the American Cancer Society, American Lung Association, and American Heart Association, hospitals are turning to the Red Cross (babysitting training), Planned Parenthood (teen sexual awareness), March of Dimes (orientation to prepared childbirth), Tuberculosis Society (smoking cessation), National Dairy Council (weight reduction), and American Dietetic Association (nutrition). Civic groups such as the Jaycees, Elks, Lions, and local chambers of commerce provide volunteers or help involve businesses in efforts to donate infant car seats and the like.

Libraries, park districts, public health departments, and other public agencies also have records of successful cooperation with hospital programs for children. PTAs often are willing to "screen" programs for school children that might prove to be controversial. In one community, the PTA collects registration money from students attending the hospital's babysitting class. Nurseries and day care centers, like schools, may be eager to be sites for children's programs. The possibilities are only as limited as the community's resources. The health educator for St. John's Hospital and Health Center, Santa Monica, CA, recommends that hospital-based educators become active in as many community groups as possible in order to learn about the wants and resources of each group. "It is hard work, but it is always mutually beneficial," she says.

### Avenues for Cooperation

Following is a sampling of the types of cooperative arrangements that have been worked out between hospitals and community groups.

- Alta View Hospital, Sandy, UT, worked with the local park district to develop its "Safety City" program.
- The Red Cross in San Pedro, CA, trained the staff of San Pedro Peninsula Hospital to teach a babysitting class.
- Planned Parenthood staff served as instructors for "Growing Up Male" and "Growing Up Female" courses for Kaiser Permanente Hospital, Martinez, CA.
- Botsford General Hospital, Farmington Hills, MI, serves as the host for various outside groups, including a program for expectant adoptive parents taught by community representatives.
- The local American Heart Association approved the CPR course taught by St. Jude Hospital, Yorba Linda, CA.
- The March of Dimes funded the development of an "Orientation to Childbirth" class for local teens. Subsequent funding allowed Freehold (NJ) Area Hospital to take the program throughout the state and to train teachers from schools outside their immediate area.
- Local Jaycees encourage members to purchase infant car seats and donate them to the hospital for rental to new parents at Freeman Hospital, Joplin, MO.
- The local Burger King gave free hamburgers to any child who said "I always wear my seat belt," as part of a promotion effort by Tod Children's Hospital, Youngstown, OH.
- The health education director at St. John's Hospital and Health Center (Santa Monica, CA) located resource people through her involvement with the American Cancer Society. She was able to use their resources to find medical students interested in working with schoolchildren.

## Needs Assessment

Without a doubt, assessing needs is one of the most important steps in planning any educational program. Only through a clear understanding of the perceived and documented needs of the target audience can a program be developed that will have the desired impact.

Assessing the needs of a target audience is not an easy task under the best of circumstances. But when that audience consists of children, many of whom can not even articulate their health needs, the problem becomes even more complex. It is therefore not surprising that many hospitals that provide health promotion programming for children have not conducted any type of formal needs assessment. Most hospitals, however, have used some kind of informal information-gathering process that has led them to select certain programs or to focus on certain health or wellness issues.

Some hospitals, on the other hand, have used native ingenuity and sound marketing practices in developing mechanisms for uncovering the health promotion needs of children and adolescents. Following are examples of a few assessment techniques that have proved successful.

## Formal Surveys, Print or Interview

There seem to be as many variations of formal surveys as there are topics to be covered, audiences to be reached, and techniques for administering them.

Formal surveys in print form can be administered by sending them to residents' homes; inserting them into local newspapers; or passing them out at health fairs, shopping centers, PTA meetings, or churches. One-on-one interview surveys, administered by trained interviewers to parents' groups, teachers, or school administrators, may be an even more successful means of eliciting information and ideas. They also may be much more expensive.

Most formal surveys are designed and administered in ways that are likely to elicit responses from adults. But when information about future children's programming is the goal, surveys targeted toward children may produce the best results. Care must be taken, of course, to make sure the reading level is appropriate to the audience; it is advisable to pilot-test any survey with a representative group of children.

Health educators at Alta View Hospital, Sandy, UT, met with school health nurses and teachers before asking them to administer a detailed health promotion survey to their students and to send it home to the pupils' parents. The preparation paid off in the form of a 98 percent response from the students and a 50 percent response from the parents (see chapter 5, "Case Study: Alta View Hospital"). Scout groups, 4-H clubs, and recreation groups also might be willing to administer surveys to their young members.

St. John's Hospital and Health Center, Santa Monica, CA, worked with the school district's public affairs department to conduct a survey of principals, vice-principals, and counselors for the hospital. Because the school district had been forced to cut back on its health education programming, the public affairs department was willing to insert questionnaires in teachers' mailboxes as a way of helping St. John's develop health classes for schoolchildren.

Following a survey of participants in a community health program, G.N. Wilcox Memorial Hospital and Health Center, Kauai, HI, instituted a program on teen depression and suicide. A separate internal assessment uncovered a need for instructing new mothers about infant car seat usage.

## Phone Surveys

Telephone surveys are, in many ways, similar to print and interview surveys. But in some instances, they allow for much more targeted queries. For example, when Freehold (NJ) Area Hospital wanted to determine whether there was a need for an asthma program for families, staff health educators called 50 to 60 school teachers to find out if asthma posed a problem for them in the classroom, and if so, how, where, and when classes should be conducted.

## Children's Involvement

Health educators at Mt. Shasta (CA) Hospital involve children, even very small children, in planning the specific content of any program directed to them. By having one or two children "walk through" the proposed class, instructors learn a great deal simply by listening to their comments and questions and by closely watching their reactions, no matter how trivial those reactions might seem to an untrained observer. Staff members feel confident that, by applying what they learn from this observation, they are addressing those aspects of the topic that are most needed and wanted by the children themselves.

## Focus Groups

Focus groups are a common technique for uncovering the feelings, attitudes, and perceptions of adults, but not many hospitals have conducted focus groups for children. Alta View Hospital, Sandy, UT, used results from two focus groups—one for children and one for their parents—to construct its large adult/children's survey. In separate groups, children and adults were asked what they thought about Alta View offering extended health promotion programming for children during the summer, what classes would be of interest, what was the likelihood of children in their family attending, where and when programs should be held, and so forth (see chapter 5, "Case Study: Alta View Hospital"). Because focus groups allow ideas to be developed through the interaction of 8 to 12 participants, they are an excellent forum for trying out new concepts.

## Questionnaires

One common mechanism used by hospitals to assess the needs of children is the questionnaire, administered to either adults or children following participation in a hospital-sponsored educational program. Often the primary thrust of the questionnaire is to evaluate the course the respondent just attended, but many have one or more additional questions about the types of programs that would be of interest to respondents in the future. Because most hospital-based programs are attended by adults, it is useful to include specific questions about children's programs in their questionnaires. Riverside Medical Center, Kankakee, IL, regularly includes on its evaluation forms a question about whether there is any interest in classes following up on the one being evaluated; through this mechanism, attendees at an adolescent weight loss clinic requested a weight loss support group.

## Interviews

Interviews need not be part of a formal survey to be useful. Periodic discussions (by phone or in person) with parents, teachers, religious leaders, scout leaders, or children can help keep health educators attuned to the issues and problems being faced by children in the community. Interviews can be used effectively before a program is implemented to determine what is needed, after a program has been conducted to identify changes that need to be made, or following a poor registration to help staff understand why the class did not appeal to the intended audience.

## Committees or Advisory Groups

Establishing a community or school health promotion committee or advisory group can help identify needs and wants of area children and also can help build strong relationships with local leaders. Juniors and seniors from Youngstown (OH) regional high schools formed a "Tod Squad" to advise Tod Children's Hospital on what students need from the hospital; they also help get students involved in the resulting health education programs. A one-time-only steering committee was useful when Dominican Santa Cruz (CA) Hospital was initially setting up its expanded health education program. Representatives included teachers, members of the chamber of commerce, senior citizens, physicians, hospital staff, and others. The hospital got good advice along with the support of area decision-makers.

## Literature Review

Periodic review of the professional and academic literature can provide information about national and regional health issues affecting children. Some hospitals find great value in keeping abreast of trends through the local and national news media and the popular press (such as women's magazines), usually in conjunction with the broader trend data available from professional journals and national statistical sources.

Newspapers in the Bergen, NJ, area were full of stories about kidnappings, sexual molestations, teen drug use, and teen suicide, so Palisades General Hospital's department of education responded with programs to address these important topics. The staff at St. Vincent's Wellness Center, Indianapolis, IN, regularly scan the leading women's magazines to identify "hot" topics.

## Records Review

School and hospital records can tell a lot about the health needs of children in the community. What kinds of problems are bringing them to the emergency room? For what illnesses are they being admitted to the hospital? Can health education help prevent any of these admissions? Do school nurses' records show any patterns of illnesses or accidents that could be addressed by prevention? Answering such questions can be as valuable as a survey.

## Patient Questionnaires

Patients, too, are in a good position to identify problems facing children that could be addressed through prevention programs. Questionnaires for inpatients and outpatients may uncover disease-related needs and wants as well as health promotion topics. Exit interviews or patient satisfaction questionnaires might be permanently altered to include health promotion needs assessment questions.

## Staff Advice

Another commonly cited technique for assessing children's health needs is listening to the suggestions and advice of hospital staff. In most cases this is an informal process. By building good relationships with staff and physicians, health educators elicit their ideas about potentially useful health promotion programming. Mental health workers at Franciscan Medical Center (Rock Island, IL) who regularly made presentations to local high schools recognized that adolescents were exhibiting high levels of stress, so they developed a stress management program for the schools.

## Community Requests

Once a hospital establishes a community health promotion program, it usually begins receiving requests for programs. The director of Bay City Hospital's Health Information Center (Chula Vista, CA) begins thinking about developing a new program "whenever I get two inquiries in close succession about the same topic." Requests for programs from community groups and individuals also can be stimulated through sending letters to community groups related to children, sending letters to teachers, or encouraging participants in the health promotion speakers' bureau to solicit requests from their audiences.

## Agency Requests

When schools, day care centers, or scout troups request specific programs, successful hospitals are fast to respond. Although it is wise to seek assurance that the suggested programs will indeed have an audience and will meet a specific need, the fact that someone takes the time to locate a community resource, place a call or write a letter, and describe a problem or desired course of action often is a strong predictor of a genuine need or want. If a program is well received and meets needs, a hospital may decide to offer it to a wider community audience.

## Program Monitoring

If assessing children's needs and wants is difficult, evaluating the effect of health promotion programs on them is even more difficult. Many hospital-based health promotion activities for children are one-shot efforts, especially those aimed at the very young, so anything more than superficial measures—such as counting attendees—may be impractical. To further complicate the matter, very young learners probably cannot fill out an evaluation form or identify whether or not their expectations have been satisfied. So hospitals have come up with a variety of ways to determine the impact of their health promotion programs on children.

### Evaluation Forms

Although many children are too young to properly fill out question-naires aimed at determining their satisfaction with and reactions to a health promotion program, forms still are a commonly used evaluation mechanism for many hospitals. Educators at Dominican Santa Cruz (CA) Hospital have found out how to effectively use evaluation forms, even with the youngest learners: they send the forms home for parents to fill out. Mothers are the source of evaluation data at St. Luke's Hospital (Davenport, IA), where questions about the sibling touch program are a part of the regular post-maternity questionnaire.

Hospitals have various uses for the results of these questionnaires. Some department directors review evaluation forms from all classes and send them to the teachers with their own suggestions. "This allows me to keep up with what is happening in a large number of classes and enables me to provide immediate feedback—both praise and ideas for improvements—to the instructors," says the community education coordinator at Community Hospital's Wellness Connection, Indianapolis, IN. Others compile the responses from all classes at the end of the year and use them in planning the following year's curriculum.

### Pre- and Post-Tests

Programs conducted in or through schools offer excellent opportunities for so-called pre- and post-tests. High school classes attending the "Orientation to Childbirth" program at Freehold (NJ) Area Hospital receive a pre-program test, prepared by the hospital and administered by the teacher during class, shortly before they attend the half-day program. A post-program test is conducted after they return to class. Teachers have been extremely cooperative about returning the results to the hospital so they can plan each presentation based on the specific attendees' prior knowledge, and so that adjustments can be made in the future if the students don't respond well to the presentation. When programs are taken into the schools, teachers are equally cooperative about conducting pre- and post-tests and sharing results with the hospital. Students in Kalamazoo (MI) schools complete pre-tests before Borgess Medical Center's "Health Factory" pays a visit. Post-tests help both hospital staff and teachers assess what degree of learning took place.

### Parent Contacts

With a large number of programs focusing on children, Dominican Santa Cruz (CA) Hospital searched for inexpensive ways to ascertain whether or not their programs were having an effect on the behavior of the attendees, even the youngest ones. So phone calls were periodically made to the parents of preschoolers enrolled in classes (see chapter 6, "Case Study: Dominican Santa Cruz Hospital"). These same calls can also serve as needs assessment tools. Letters mailed to parents of attendees or sent home with children can serve the same purposes.

### Tracking Census

A few programs, such as presurgical orientations, lend themselves to using census data as a direct form of evaluation. At MedCenter One (Bismarck, ND) the presurgical program is open to all children, regardless of which hospital their parents plan to use. Education department staff monitor the number of children from this program who actually check into MedCenter One. Recently, one child who attended the class—which features a life-sized bear mascot named "Meddy Bear"— became so disheartened when he learned he was not being admitted to "Meddy Bear's hospital" that his mother switched to MedCenter One. Staff at the Center for Sports Medicine and Health Fitness, St. Francis Medical Center, Peoria, IL, track the number of admissions and surgeries that are a direct result of individuals' using the center.

### Tracking Community Statistics

Some indication of the impact of programs designed to address such social problems as suicide, kidnapping, and child abuse can be obtained by tracking local statistics. Certainly no one expects to see a dramatic reduction in problems as soon as a hospital offers a related health promotion class—no cause-and-effect relationship can be attributed to just one class, or possibly even to a series—but such figures can provide one additional piece of information for the evaluation puzzle.

## Counting Attendees

Although they are not necessarily an indicator of program effectiveness, attendance statistics certainly offer a quick assessment of a program's popularity, especially if the program included several
successive sessions. Was attendance at the last session as high as at
the first? Or, if the class is repeated frequently, does word of mouth
increase attendance? Many program directors state that this is the
only type of evaluation data required by their administration. At the
Toledo (OH) Hospital, staff contact former participants to learn why
they haven't reregistered. These calls have become an excellent
source of information about new competitors in the community,
changes in school activities, and other changes in the market.

## Staff Observations

Stress management and nutrition classes (when conducted for an
audience that uses a central cafeteria) lend themselves to evaluation
by observation of health habits. Do attendees exhibit a decrease in
stress-related behaviors such as nail-biting, sleeplessness, or fidget-
ing in class? Do they select more "healthy" foods? Even long-term
results from a weight loss program can be tracked to some extent
through observations of whether the attendees appear to have gained
back weight, maintained their weight, or continued to reduce their
weight.

## Reconvening Classes

Couples who took part in St. Jude Hospital and Rehabilitation Center's
prepared childbirth classes in Fullerton, CA, are invited to get reac-
quainted and to meet each other's babies. During the evening, they
are given information about infant stimulation and growth and
development. A discussion of whether or not the childbirth class
proved to be useful could provide excellent feedback for the instructors. Girls who complete the babysitting class offered by Community
Hospital, Indianapolis, IN, are invited to a swim party at the end of
the summer. Inasmuch as they probably have used their new babysitting skills during the summer, this nonthreatening environment could
produce a good evaluation discussion.

# Publicity and Promotion

Even the best health promotion program will not generate an audience
unless people know about it. Publicity and promotion are keys to the
success of many hospital-based programs for children. The use of certain vehicles for promoting programs for and about children and teens
seems to be almost commonplace among hospitals—flyers and
brochures describing offerings, catalogs, press releases sent to

newspapers and local broadcast outlets, public service messages, and letters to key audiences such as physicians and school health nurses. Other less frequently used but still effective means of communication include paid ads, billboards, special luncheons, physician referral forms, identifiable mascots, and co-sponsorship of programs by communications media or community agencies.

But before discussing how some of these methods have been used, it is important to consider the selection of the right channels for distributing print materials.

## Distribution Channels

The fact that attractive brochures or catalogs have been designed in no way guarantees that they will reach the intended audience. Careful thought must be given to who receives them and how.

### Mailings

Information aimed at children or their parents will have the greatest impact if mailings are carefully targeted rather than sent, for example, to all homes within certain zip codes. Lists of attendees at previous classes for children or parents are an excellent base for a mailing list, as are lists of attendees at health fairs geared to youngsters and membership lists from scout troops or church youth groups.

Marlborough (MA) Hospital has had great success in building a mailing list of attendees at its "Well Doll Clinic" (see chapter 4, "Community Health Promotion Programs for Children and Teens": New Approaches to Tried-and-True Topics) and using it to publicize other activities for children, especially little girls. Members of PTAs, teachers, and pediatricians are examples of other groups that may generate a high payoff from mailings.

### Other Channels

Schools sometimes will send flyers home with children if the right bridges have been built with teachers and administrators. Some schools will even reproduce the materials for students. Others want brochures packaged into groups of 25 or 30, depending on the average size of their classes. Physicians, especially pediatricians, may be willing to hand out catalogs to parents during pre-school physical exams. Libraries, supermarkets, boosters clubs, and churches also are popular distribution points for materials.

## Other Promotional Vehicles

Many hospitals have gone well beyond the usual print and mail promotional materials. Following are a few ideas to stimulate thinking about what avenues might be effective under specific community circumstances.

### Telephone Contacts

Direct telephone contact is one way to use friends of the hospital or members of a community advisory group. Give them advance information about new offerings for youngsters and ask them to tell their neighbors and members of their groups (churches, PTAs, scouts, and so forth).

### Radio and Television Shows

In addition to press releases and public service announcements, appearances on local talk or news shows will reach a big audience. In order to have the greatest chance for success, these should be keyed to a major offering ("25 new summer programs for children and adolescents!"), a catchy program ("Surviving with Working Parents"), or a subject with current news value (teen suicide). A health educator teamed with an expert on the topic will have a good chance of getting air time.

### Paid Ads

Hospitals that have a history of offering health promotion programs for a young audience sometimes find it difficult to generate news or feature coverage in the local media year after year. So some place paid ads designed to publicize their classes. Freehold (NJ) Area Hospital obtained a small grant from the local American Lung Association to purchase ad space for its family asthma program, which used ALA materials.

### Features and News Stories

Newspapers, radio, and television report on upcoming programs, especially if they feature timely topics (suicide or kidnap prevention) and they also may cover the class itself—a wellness camp, for example. Sometimes a children's health promotion program may even become a news story. In Indianapolis, IN, a youngster saved the life of an infant because of the skills she learned through a babysitting class sponsored by a local hospital. Her heroism was covered extensively by the local newspaper, and the class got some excellent publicity.

### Billboards

Hospitals are beginning to use billboards as part of their overall campaigns to establish a clear "identity" for the institution and keep their name in front of the public. A few, like Alta View Hospital, Sandy, UT, have had success in using billboards to publicize expanded children's programming. Billboard companies may even donate space or offer it at a discounted rate.

*Luncheons*

Special luncheons or breakfasts (especially for busy physicians) provide not only an opportunity to introduce children's programs to community decision-makers but also the opportunity for these leaders to make suggestions for expanding or refining the program. Invited guests might include school nurses, health education teachers, religious leaders, church auxiliary members, civic club presidents, youth group leaders, and so forth. Information about the hospital's programs for children can be integrated into other ongoing luncheons or meetings, such as monthly auxiliary meetings or regular breakfast meetings for hospital trustees.

*Talks to Community Groups*

Hospitals should provide a list of new program offerings to everyone involved in their speakers' bureau, with information about the community and school programs available for children and families. This will keep speakers up to date, get current information to the community, and help keep speakers involved as an important part of the children's program. Some may even give speeches to local social and civic groups on child-related topics that tie in to new classes.

*Mascots*

Several hospitals have developed special characters or mascots for their children's activities, both in the hospital and in the community.

Tod Children's Hospital, Youngstown, OH, uses a series of characters called the "Tod Squad" on all its materials for children, and young patients are invited to become members of the "Tod Squad's Get-Well Team." These same characters are seen in action when the hospital takes its "Mini-Hospital" to a local shopping mall (see chapter 4, "Creative Approaches to Keeping Children Healthy"— Tried-and-True Programs).

Cute and cuddly "Meddy Bear" comes in many sizes at Med-Center One, Bismarck, ND, including several life-size versions that walk and talk. This mascot was introduced at a public birthday party that attracted over 500 people, and has become a staple in hospital-based school and presurgical orientation programs. A nurse dressed in a "Meddy Bear" costume also appears before community groups, and is ready to help out in the Children's Health Center and in same-day surgery if a child becomes frightened or if staff members cannot communicate effectively with a patient (costumes are kept handy in key places). To carry the theme further, each child admitted to the pediatric unit receives a twelve-inch "Meddy Bear," and when he or she gets a shot or a bandage, so does the mascot. "Meddy Bear" is used extensively on materials and brochures, generates a great deal of positive publicity, and has come to be associated with MedCenter One by children all over the Bismarck area.

*Cosponsorship of Events*

An almost certain way to generate publicity is to involve a newspaper or radio or TV station in cosponsoring an event. Hazel Hawkins Memorial Hospital, Hollister, CA, is one of many institutions that has worked with a local newspaper to promote a "fun run." In Hollister, adults run or walk five miles, and children under 12 are invited to run or walk one mile, for good health. To avoid pressuring young runners into pushing themselves too hard, no trophies are awarded in the youth category, but everyone who finishes gets a blue ribbon.

## Fees and Budget

Because most hospitals integrate programs for children with programs for adults, it is difficult to establish budget levels for children's programs. Those hospitals that attempt to budget for childrens' programming and to determine what level of revenue is necessary to cover associated expenses often include such direct costs as salaries and fees, materials, promotion, supplies, and advertising costs. Office and classroom space, capital expenditures such as depreciation on equipment and plant, and allocation of overhead and shared services also may be budgeted against the program.

Different patterns can be seen in the way hospitals handle such areas as deciding whether programs need to generate revenue, setting fees (if any are to be charged), and finding funding for children's programs.

### Charging Fees

Although it is not known whether most hospitals currently offer children's programs for free or charge a fee, it does appear that the following guidelines generally apply:

- Most school programs are offered without charge.
- Most hospital orientation programs and presurgical orientation programs are offered without charge, even when other activities for children require a fee.
- Hospitals with a small number of offerings are likely to provide all programs free, regardless of the content.
- Individual programs are often provided free of charge when they are provided primarily as a marketing device for a hospital service (a sports medicine program designed to acquaint the community with a new sports medicine department) or to make potential patients aware of the expertise of local physicians (an eating disorders lecture presented by a doctor specializing in this problem).
- Most hospitals that do charge for classes for children attempt to set fees as low as possible. One institution's fees range from

$7, for a 2-hour class, to $25, which covers a whole family for six 1½-hour classes. At another hospital, fees go from $5 for a 2-hour class to $60 for a 12-week weight management class. Five days at a wellness camp may be priced as low as $40, including lunches.

- Some hospitals set fees to cover the cost of instructors and/or classroom costs.
- Hospitals that generate significant amounts of revenue (see Revenue Generation, below) are likely to do so through volume (high attendance) rather than through high fees.
- Some hospitals that have traditionally offered children's programs free are considering switching to nominal fees because of the pressure on their departments to cover at least some expenses.

## Revenue Generation

The vast majority of hospitals see programming for children as an integral part of their overall health promotion effort and as a manifestation of their commitment to fostering a healthy community; thus they have no specific goals to cover expenses or generate a profit. However, two hospitals with extensive programming for children and teens are illustrative of the growing number of institutions that have identified specific revenue-generating goals for their community health education departments.

- By offering as many as 100 classes per quarter, paying teachers a percentage of the revenue they generate rather than a straight fee, and by "operating on a shoestring," Dominican Santa Cruz (CA) Hospital has paid back its initial start-up grant of $20,000 and has generated an additional $20,000 profit. The department's goal is to make an increasing profit in order to help offset hospital expenses.
- Activities at Alta View Hospital, Sandy, UT, also have accelerated in the last two years; children's programs generated income of $36,000 in 1984. Alta View has experienced a 700 percent increase in revenue in two years, and hopes soon to cover all its direct expenses.

Additional details about how both these hospitals budget and generate revenue can be found in chapters 5 and 6.

## Sources of Funding

Although in some hospitals fees offset some expenses of presenting school and community health promotion programs for children, the prevailing source of funding for such activities is the hospitals themselves. But other sources of funding are being tapped.

### Donations

In addition to financial donations and volunteer help, hospitals often seek materials or services from local donors. At St. Jude Hospital,

Yorba Linda, CA, concerned citizens, corporations, and professional associations donated mannequins for the CPR "Heartsavers" class designed for 9-to-18-year-olds. In Joplin, MO, Freeman Hospital accepts infant care seats donated by businesses and individuals, then rents them to new parents. The list of potential donors is almost endless—voluntary groups, civic groups, women's clubs, parents groups, businesses, trade associations, and so on.

Botsford General Hospital, Farmington Hills, MI, has found that individuals, businesses, and service groups are more willing to donate money to support a specific activity, such as an infant and toddlers car seat rental program, than to donate general funds to underwrite wellness efforts. Once donors have had a positive experience with the wellness program, Botsford hopes they will become the basis for a wellness fund-raising network.

*Contracts*

Hospitals are increasingly likely to write contracts with schools or other groups to whom they offer children's health promotion programs. This practice is probably most common today in the area of sports medicine. Fees charged for sports-related services offered to schools are designed to cover costs and, in some cases, to generate extra revenue for the hospital. Fees usually are bundled under one contract and cover a season or a full school year. Contracts usually contain information about the services to be rendered, the time frame involved, and the number of children covered. For example, a contract might specify that the hospital will provide (1) game coverage by a physician or a trainer for the basketball season, (2) preseason physicals for the entire swim team, and (3) a physician to be available for one hour after all football games for evaluation of injuries. Contracts also might include clauses providing discounts for other sports-related services to students and their families if students are covered by the school's contract.

*Grants*

Money in the form of grants is available from government agencies (local, state, and federal), from voluntary agencies, sometimes from local businesses, and potentially from almost any source that is interested in children or in a particular topic. Martin Luther King Jr. Hospital, Los Angeles, CA, has received numerous grants from the state to develop special materials addressing current needs for minority teens, such as teen pregnancy. The March of Dimes funded an "Orientation to Childbirth" class for teens through Freehold (NJ) Area Hospital.

Grant monies also may be available from groups associated with the hospital. Dominican Santa Cruz (CA) Hospital received a start-up grant in the form of a loan to expand its health education program from the hospital's foundation. The Hospital and Medical Staff Guild gave Queen of the Valley Hospital, West Covina, (CA) a grant to develop its "Home Accident Prevention Project for Young Children" program, which trained 20 preschool teachers to educate parents about home accident prevention.

*Sale of Materials*

Once an investment has been made in a good program or in specialized materials, hospitals can sell them to other institutions or groups. A series of videotapes with such titles as "The Amazing Body," "Drugs? The Choice is Crystal Clear," and "Divorce: Kids in the Middle," were developed and made available free of charge to all hospitals in the Samaritan Health Services system in Arizona, as well as to local groups in communities surrounding SHS hospitals. Now that the materials have been deemed a success, SHS plans to sell them to other groups.

## Summary

The tasks involved in managing a health promotion program for children are generally similar from hospital to hospital. How each one handles market analysis, publicity and promotion, educational review, and the numerous other aspects of program management, is dependent on the community the hospital serves, the hospital's mission as reflected in its goals for children's health programming, and the resources available in the hospital and the community. Making a health promotion program work, however, is mainly dependent on the perseverance and creativity of hospital staff as they gather large amounts of data, examine them, synthesize them, and ultimately turn them into a product that meets the needs of the community and the hospital.

American Hospital Publishing, Inc.
211 East Chicago Avenue
Chicago, Illinois 60611

Catalog no. 070189

ISBN 0-939450-9